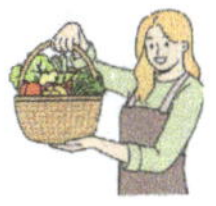

# TABLE OF CONTENT

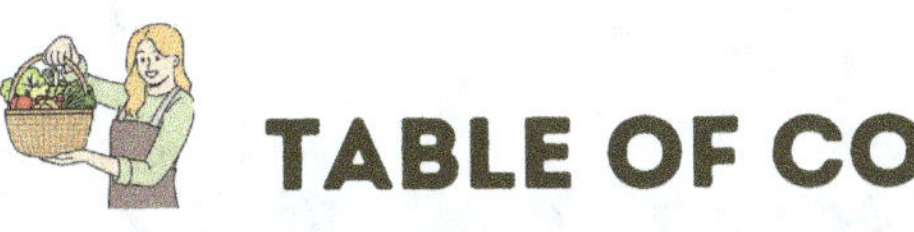

# TABLE OF CONTENT

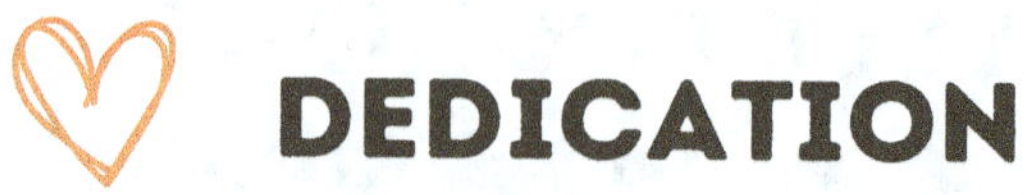

# DEDICATION

To all the Jennifers of the world,

This book is dedicated to you—the busy mothers, the hardworking professionals, the determined individuals who have faced the ups and downs of weight loss journeys. To my own mother, whose strength and resilience have always been my guiding light, and to every person who has ever felt the frustration of yo-yo dieting and the emotional toll of restrictive diets.

Remember, you are not alone in this journey. The path to weight loss and self-love is not a straight line, but a series of steps, each one bringing you closer to your goals. Embrace the process, celebrate the small victories, and be kind to yourself along the way.

Intermittent fasting is more than just a method for losing weight; it's a lifestyle that can bring balance, health, and happiness. Believe in your ability to succeed, and know that with the right mindset and support, you can achieve lasting change.

Never give up on yourself. You are worth the effort, the time, and the love. Here's to a healthier, happier you.

With all my heart,

ONEMIRACLE PUBLISHING

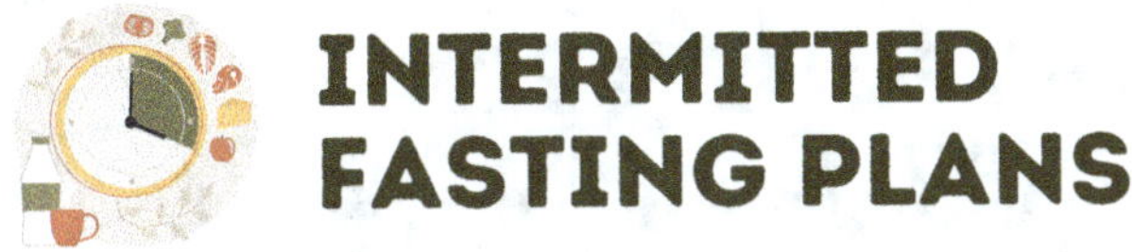

# INTERMITTED FASTING PLANS

| PLAN | OVERVIEW | HOW | TIPS |
|---|---|---|---|
| **12/12** | Fasting Period: 12 hours<br><br>Eating Window: 12 hours | Fast for 12 hours each day, such as from 7 PM to 7 AM. Eat during the remaining 12 hours.<br><br>This method is a great starting point for beginners. | Gradually adjust your eating and fasting times to ease into the routine.<br><br>Stay hydrated with water, herbal teas, and black coffee during fasting periods.<br><br>Focus on nutrient-dense foods during your eating window. |
| **16/18** | Fasting Period: 16 hours<br><br>Eating Window: 8 hours | Fast for 16 hours each day, such as from 8 PM to 12 PM (the next day)<br><br>Eat during the 8-hour window, typically including two to three meals. | Start with a 12-hour fast and gradually increase to 16 hours.<br><br>Drink plenty of water and non-caloric beverages during the fasting period.<br><br>Plan your meals to include a balance of proteins, healthy fats, and whole grains. |

Intermittent fasting (IF) is a popular eating pattern that alternates between periods of fasting and eating. It's not about what you eat, but when you eat. This guide will introduce you to various intermittent fasting plans, from beginner-friendly to more advanced methods, and provide tips on how to follow them effectively.

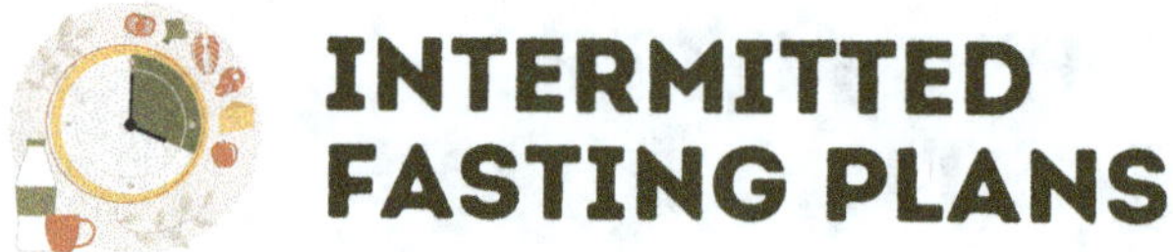

# INTERMITTED FASTING PLANS

| PLAN | OVERVIEW | HOW | TIPS |
|---|---|---|---|
| **18/6** | Fasting Period: 18 hours<br><br>Eating Window: 6 hours | Fast for 18 hours each day, such as from 6 PM to 12 PM (the next day).<br><br>Eat during the 6-hour window, typically including two meals. | Gradually extend your fasting period from 16 to 18 hours.<br><br>Stay hydrated and consider adding electrolytes to your water.<br><br>Focus on nutrient-dense foods to ensure you get enough nutrients in a shorter eating window. |
| **20/4** | Fasting Period: 20 hours<br><br>Eating Window: 4 hours | Fast for 20 hours each day, such as from 8 PM to 4 PM (the next day).<br><br>Eat during the 4-hour window, typically including one large meal and a small snack. | Start with shorter fasting periods and gradually increase to 20 hours.<br><br>Plan your meals ahead to avoid impulsive eating.<br><br>Focus on high-quality, nutrient-dense foods to maximize the benefits. |

Intermittent fasting (IF) is a popular eating pattern that alternates between periods of fasting and eating. It's not about what you eat, but when you eat. This guide will introduce you to various intermittent fasting plans, from beginner-friendly to more advanced methods, and provide tips on how to follow them effectively.

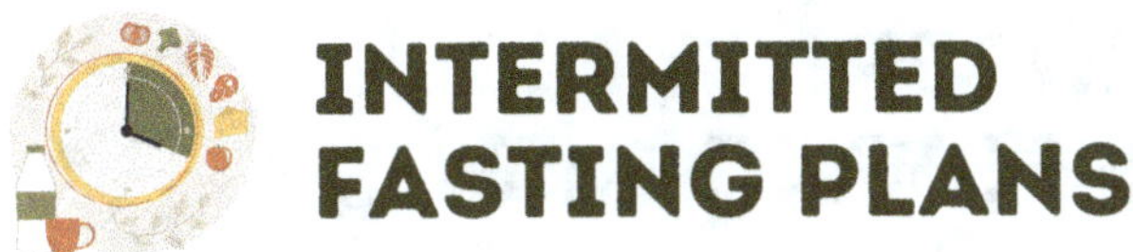

# INTERMITTED FASTING PLANS

| PLAN | OVERVIEW | HOW | TIPS |
| --- | --- | --- | --- |
| **5:2** | Fasting Period: 2 non-consecutive days per week<br><br>Eating Window: 5 days per week | On fasting days, consume only 500–600 calories.<br><br>Eat normally on the other five days of the week. | Choose fasting days that fit your schedule and avoid consecutive fasting days.<br><br>Plan low-calorie, nutrient-dense meals for fasting days.<br><br>Stay hydrated and consider light physical activity on fasting days. |
| **Alternate Day Fasting (ADF)** | Fasting Period: Every other day<br><br>Eating Window: Alternate day | Fast every other day, consuming only 500–600 calories on fasting days.<br><br>Eat normally on non-fasting days. | Start with a modified version, such as 500–600 calories on fasting days, before attempting full fasting.<br><br>Stay hydrated and listen to your body's signals.<br><br>Plan your meals to ensure you get enough nutrients on both fasting and non-fasting days. |

Intermittent fasting (IF) is a popular eating pattern that alternates between periods of fasting and eating. It's not about what you eat, but when you eat. This guide will introduce you to various intermittent fasting plans, from beginner-friendly to more advanced methods, and provide tips on how to follow them effectively.

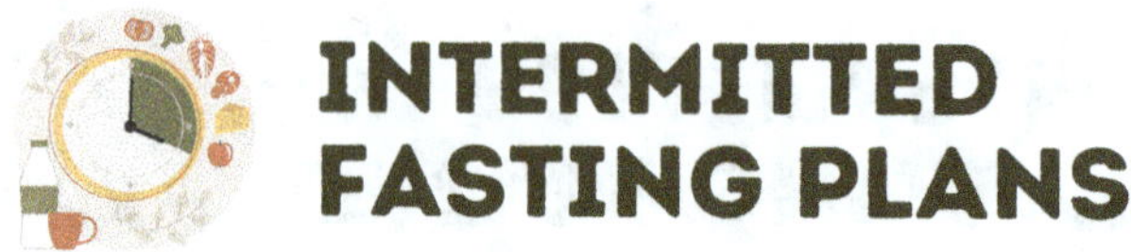

# INTERMITTED FASTING PLANS

| PLAN | OVERVIEW | HOW | TIPS |
|---|---|---|---|
| **Eat Stop Eat** | Fasting Period: 24 hours once or twice a week | Fast for 24 hours once or twice a week, such as from dinner one day to dinner the next day.<br><br>Eat normally on non-fasting days. | Start with shorter fasting periods and gradually increase to 24 hours.<br><br>Stay hydrated with water, herbal teas, and black coffee.<br><br>Plan your meals to ensure you get enough nutrients on non-fasting days. |

## GENERAL TIPS

**Stay Hydrated:** Drink plenty of water and non-caloric beverages during fasting periods to stay hydrated and manage hunger.

**Listen to Your Body:** Pay attention to hunger cues and adjust your fasting schedule as needed.

**Focus on Nutrient-Dense Foods:** Prioritize whole foods, lean proteins, healthy fats, and plenty of fruits and vegetables during your eating windows.

**Plan Your Meals:** Prepare meals in advance to avoid impulsive eating and ensure you get the necessary nutrients.

**Be Patient:** Give your body time to adjust to the new eating pattern. It may take a few weeks to see significant results.

**Consult a Healthcare Professional:** Before starting any fasting regimen, especially if you have underlying health conditions, consult with a healthcare provider to ensure it's safe for you.

By understanding and choosing the right intermittent fasting plan for your lifestyle and goals, you can effectively harness the benefits of this eating pattern for weight loss, improved health, and overall well-being.

# CHAPTER 1: EMBARKING ON THE INTERMITTED FASTING JOURNEY

Meet Jennifer, a bustling mother of two, juggling a demanding job and household chores. Like many, Jennifer had battled with her weight for years, adhering to various traditional diets that seemed promising at first but ultimately led to disappointment. She'd lose some pounds, only to see them come creeping back with a vengeance—a disheartening cycle often referred to as "yo-yo dieting." Frustrated and feeling defeated, she stumbled upon intermittent fasting while browsing through health forums late one night, and it changed everything for her. The flexibility and simplicity of intermittent fasting appealed to her hectic lifestyle, and to her surprise, the results were not just quick but sustainable.

The struggle Jennifer faced isn't unique. Obesity is on the rise globally, creating a public health crisis. According to recent statistics, nearly 40% of adults in the United States are obese, and this number has been climbing steadily over the past few decades. Maintaining weight loss has become an increasingly challenging endeavor, compounded by modern life's demands and the constant bombardment of unhealthy food choices (Contreras et al., 2019).

Traditional diets often set people up for failure because they focus on intense restriction.

Whether it's low-carb or low-fat, these diets usually emphasize eliminating entire food groups or drastically slashing calorie intake, leading to what experts call the deprivation mindset. Many of us have experienced that gnawing sense of being starved for something—whether it's a favorite treat or simply enough calories to feel full—which eventually leads to binge eating or giving up on the diet entirely. This is where the frustration of yo-yo dieting kicks in, leaving individuals feeling like they're stuck in a never-ending loop of gaining and losing weight.

The emotional toll of traditional diets shouldn't be underestimated either. People often report feelings of guilt and shame when they stray from their rigid eating plans. This negative self-talk exacerbates stress and may induce emotional eating as a coping mechanism. Further complicating matters, restrictive dieting can slow down your metabolism, making it even harder to lose weight the next time you try

.

Intermittent fasting offers a refreshing departure from these restrictive methods. Rather than focusing on what you eat, it zeros in on when you eat. By designating specific periods for eating and fasting, this approach naturally reduces calorie intake and allows your body time to reset. Research shows that intermittent fasting can improve metabolic health, reduce insulin resistance, and even promote longevity. It's less about cutting out your favorite foods and more about finding a rhythm that works harmoniously with your life.

Before diving headfirst into intermittent fasting, it's essential to cultivate the right mindset—a crucial element for long-term success frequently overlooked in weight-loss endeavors. A positive and resilient mindset can make all the difference. Without it, you're likely to fall back into the traps of yo-yo dieting and emotional eating . But how do you foster such a mindset?

- Focus on how foods make you feel rather than labeling them as 'good' or 'bad.' Pay attention to energy levels, mood, and overall well-being after consuming different foods.

- Emphasize addition instead of subtraction. Rather than fixating on what you should eliminate, focus on adding nutrient-rich foods like vegetables, fruits, and lean proteins. This shift creates a sense of abundance rather than scarcity.

- Challenge negative self-talk. Recognize when you're being overly critical of yourself. Instead, celebrate small victories, like drinking an extra glass of water or choosing a healthy snack.

- Harness the power of self-efficacy—believe in your ability to succeed. Track your progress, and make adjustments as needed. Pay attention to triggers that might lead to unhealthy habits and develop strategies to address them.

- Cultivate a growth mindset. Viewing setbacks as learning opportunities rather than failures helps maintain momentum. Understand that weight loss is a journey with ups and downs.

One thing Jennifer noted during her initial attempts at intermittent fasting was the importance of support and accountability. Having a community or even just a buddy trying the same approach can significantly boost your chances of sticking with it. Joining a group, whether online or in-person, where you can share experiences and insights can provide invaluable motivation.

Intermittent fasting also aligns well with sustainable lifestyle changes recommended by experts. Dr. Katie Hanisee emphasizes the importance of adopting long-term changes rather than seeking quick fixes. These changes should include regular physical activity and balanced nutrition tailored to individual needs. Seeking professional guidance from registered dietitians or mental health experts specializing in weight loss can further bolster your efforts.

Let's not forget the significance of social and environmental factors in the weight loss journey. Our surroundings and social circles can heavily influence our eating habits and overall health behaviors. It's beneficial to create an environment that supports your goals. This might mean having healthier food options readily available or seeking out friends who share your health aspirations.

Integration is key here. Intermittent fasting isn't a standalone solution but part of a broader strategy encompassing diet, exercise, mindset, and social support. When considered collectively, these elements can help break the cycle of yo-yo dieting and pave the way for lasting weight loss and improved health.

Jennifer's story is a testament to the transformative power of intermittent fasting when coupled with the right mindset and support systems. Her journey underscores the necessity of moving beyond restrictive diets and embracing a holistic approach that values both personal freedom and social responsibility. With evidence-based strategies in place, attainable and sustainable weight loss isn't just a dream—it's a realistic goal within reach for anyone willing to take that first step.

By addressing the root causes of weight gain and implementing supportive structures, we can create an environment conducive to real, lasting change. Whether you're looking to shed pounds to feel better, improve your health, or achieve a specific body goal, intermittent fasting presents a flexible and evidence-driven option worth considering. The road ahead may have its challenges, but armed with the right tools and mindset, you too can achieve your weight loss goals.

## A sustainable solution

Many people feel frustrated and defeated when it comes to weight loss, especially after trying countless diets that seem impossible to maintain. The thought of giving up your favorite foods can be disheartening, and the endless cycle of losing weight only to gain it back again takes an emotional toll. It's important to find a method that's sustainable in the long term—one that fits seamlessly into a busy lifestyle without demanding excessive meal prep or rigid restrictions.

Intermittent fasting has emerged as a promising approach due to its flexibility and practicality. This method doesn't require you to count every calorie or eliminate the foods you love. Instead, it focuses on when you eat rather than what you eat. The principle behind intermittent fasting is simple: limit your eating to specific periods and allow your body to spend more time in a fasted state. This approach can offer numerous benefits, particularly for those struggling to juggle weight loss with other life demands.

To understand why intermittent fasting could be the key to successful weight loss, it's helpful to look at the science. Research indicates that being in a fasted state promotes beneficial cellular processes. When you're not consuming food, your body switches from burning glucose to burning stored fats. This switch not only aids in weight loss but also enhances cellular repair mechanisms and increases insulin sensitivity, making it easier to maintain a healthy weight over time.
But beyond the science, real-life success stories resonate the most. Take Jim Caldwell, who once weighed 352 pounds and struggled with ineffective diet attempts. After adopting intermittent fasting and

focusing on eating one healthy meal a day, he successfully shed over half his body weight, reaching a stable 164 pounds. Caldwell's journey underscores how approachable and sustainable intermittent fasting can be, even for those who have faced repeated setbacks with traditional dieting methods.

It's crucial, however, to understand that not all forms of intermittent fasting will work equally well for everyone. For instance, a common protocol like the 16/8 method—where you fast for 16 hours and eat during an 8-hour window—may suit many people. However, the results can vary depending on individual lifestyles and metabolic rates. What's essential is finding the right balance that aligns with your daily schedule and nutritional needs.

Scientific studies bolster the credibility of this method. For example, research published by Harvard Health Publishing emphasizes that intermittent fasting can lead to modest yet significant weight loss. One study noted that participants practicing time-restricted eating lost an average of 18 pounds over a year, comparable to the weight loss achieved through traditional calorie restriction. More importantly, these results were obtained without participants feeling overly deprived or restricted, making it easier to stick with the plan in the long run.

So how do you get started? Here are some steps to help you incorporate intermittent fasting into your routine effectively:

- Begin with a manageable fasting schedule. Start with a 12-hour fast—say from 7 PM to 7 AM—and gradually increase the fasting period to 14 or 16 hours as your body adjusts.

- Ensure you stay hydrated. Drink plenty of water during your fasting window and consider herbal teas or black coffee if you need something warm.

- Focus on nutrient-dense foods during your eating window. Prioritize whole foods, lean proteins, healthy fats, and plenty of vegetables to provide your body with essential nutrients.

- Listen to your body. Pay attention to hunger cues and avoid the temptation to overeat during your eating window, which can negate the benefits of fasting.

- Incorporate physical activity. Pairing intermittent fasting with regular exercise, particularly resistance training, can help preserve muscle mass while you lose fat, enhancing overall metabolic health.

While intermittent fasting can offer a viable pathway to sustainable weight loss, it isn't a one-size-fits-all solution. Some individuals, such as those with diabetes, pregnant women, or people with eating disorders, should approach fasting cautiously or seek alternative methods. Consulting a healthcare professional before starting any new diet regimen is always wise. Furthermore, it's vital to remember that the quantity and quality of food still matter within your eating window. Binge-eating unhealthy foods because they fit within your time frame will undermine your efforts. Aim for balanced meals that nourish your body and support your weight loss goals.

Ultimately, intermittent fasting offers a flexible and evidence-backed approach to weight management that can adapt to various lifestyles and preferences. It allows you to enjoy your favorite foods in moderation while fostering a healthier relationship with eating patterns. By aligning with our body's natural rhythms and reducing the burden of constant meal planning, intermittent fasting simplifies the weight loss journey, making it a realistic and enduring choice for achieving and maintaining a healthy weight.

This pragmatic approach, underpinned by solid scientific research and reinforced by inspiring personal success stories, provides hope and encouragement. With intermittent fasting, you don't have to navigate the exhausting maze of fad diets and restrictive plans. Instead, you can embrace a smarter, more sustainable way to reach your weight loss goals while enjoying a balanced, satisfying life.

## Taking the first step

In this chapter, we delved into how intermittent fasting can set the stage for successful weight loss. By exploring Jennifer's story, we've highlighted the common frustrations and setbacks many face with raditional diets, particularly the cycle of yo-yo dieting. We've shown that focusing on when you eat, rather than just what you eat, can make a significant difference in achieving sustainable results.

Returning to the struggles shared by many, like Jennifer's initial despair, we recognize the emotional and physical toll of restrictive diets. Our current approach advocates for intermittent fasting as a more realistic and less restrictive method, aligning well with busy lifestyles and long-term health goals.

However, there are concerns to consider. Not every form of intermittent fasting suits everyone. Individual needs vary, and it's crucial to find a method that fits seamlessly into one's daily routine. Moreover, consulting healthcare professionals before starting any new diet regimen ensures safety and effectiveness, especially for those with pre-existing health conditions. On a broader scale, adopting intermittent fasting alongside other lifestyle changes—like regular exercise and a nutritious diet—can potentially transform public health. If more people shift from fad diets to sustainable approaches, we might see a decrease in obesity rates and related health issues, paving the way for a healthier society.

Remember that weight loss is a journey, one that can be made less daunting with intermittent fasting. It offers a flexible, science-backed way to meet your goals without feeling deprived. With the right mindset and support system, you're not just embarking on another diet—you're embracing a new way of living that values balance and well-being. The road ahead may have its ups and downs, but with intermittent fasting, lasting change is within reach. So, why not take that first step and see where it leads?

# CHAPTER 2: UNDERSTANDING THE SCIENCE AND BENEFITS BEHIND FASTING

Intermittent fasting has gained significant traction in recent years as a powerful tool for weight management and overall health optimization. While its effectiveness for sustainable weight loss is well-documented, the benefits of this dietary approach extend far beyond the realm of shedding excess pounds. In this chapter, we will delve into the multifaceted advantages of intermittent fasting, exploring its impact on metabolism, cognitive function, and longevity.

## Weight Loss and Metabolic Health

One of the primary draws of intermittent fasting is its ability to promote weight loss in a sustainable and natural manner. By creating a calorie deficit during fasting periods, the body is forced to tap into its stored energy reserves, primarily in the form of fat. This process, known as fat oxidation, not only facilitates weight loss but also enhances overall metabolic health.

During fasting, the body experiences a cascade of hormonal changes that prime it for efficient fat burning. Insulin levels decrease, allowing the body to access and utilize stored fats more readily.

Additionally, intermittent fasting has been shown to

Increase the production of growth hormone and norepinephrine, both of which contribute to enhanced fat metabolism and preservation of lean muscle mass. Unlike traditional calorie-restrictive diets, intermittent fasting will allow you to experience sustained weight loss results without the risk of significant muscle loss. By strategically timing nutrient intake, the body can maintain its lean muscle mass while selectively targeting stubborn fat deposits. This unique advantage not only supports a leaner physique but also contributes to a higher metabolic rate, further aiding in long-term weight management.

Understanding the science behind weight loss during fasting periods can empower individuals to make informed dietary choices. By recognizing the body's natural ability to burn fat for energy, individuals can embrace intermittent fasting as a sustainable and effective approach to achieving their desired body composition goals.

## Metabolic Health and Insulin Sensitivity

Beyond its weight loss benefits, intermittent fasting has been shown to have a profound impact on overall metabolic health. One of the key mechanisms underlying this effect is the improvement in insulin sensitivity.

During fasting periods, the body's insulin levels naturally decrease, allowing cells to become more responsive to the hormone. This enhanced insulin sensitivity not only aids in better blood sugar control but also reduces the risk of developing insulin resistance, a precursor to type 2 diabetes.

Furthermore, intermittent fasting has been linked to increased fat oxidation and improved mitochondrial function, both of which contribute to a more efficient metabolism. By optimizing metabolic processes, intermittent fasting can support weight loss efforts while simultaneously reducing inflammation and oxidative stress within the body.

Implementing intermittent fasting strategies can have a profound impact on overall metabolic health, potentially lowering the risk of chronic diseases associated with metabolic dysfunction, such as obesity, cardiovascular disease, and certain types of cancer. By promoting a healthier metabolism and reducing inflammation, intermittent fasting offers a powerful tool for long-term well-being and disease prevention.

## Cognitive Function and Brain Health

The benefits of intermittent fasting extend beyond physical health and weight management. Emerging research suggests that this dietary approach may also have a positive impact on cognitive function and brain health.

Studies have linked intermittent fasting to improved focus, memory retention, and overall cognitive performance. This enhancement is thought to be mediated by the cellular repair process known as autophagy, which is activated during fasting periods.

Autophagy plays a crucial role in removing damaged or dysfunctional cellular components, including those in the brain. By promoting this process, intermittent fasting may contribute to the maintenance of healthy brain cells and potentially reduce the risk of neurodegenerative diseases like Alzheimer's and Parkinson's.

Additionally, intermittent fasting has been associated with increased production of brain-derived neurotrophic factor (BDNF), a protein that supports the growth and survival of neurons. This mechanism may further contribute to improved cognitive function and overall brain health.

By exploring the holistic benefits of intermittent fasting beyond physical health, individuals can be inspired to adopt a sustainable lifestyle approach that supports both mental and physical well-being. Embracing intermittent fasting as a long-term practice may not only aid in weight management but also potentially enhance cognitive performance and protect against age-related cognitive decline.

## Longevity and Healthy Aging

One of the most intriguing areas of research surrounding intermittent fasting is its potential impact on longevity and healthy aging. While the mechanisms are still being explored, several studies have suggested that intermittent fasting may activate cellular pathways that promote longevity and delay the onset of age-related diseases.

At the cellular level, intermittent fasting has been shown to influence gene expression and activate pathways involved in cellular protection and repair. These pathways play a crucial role in mitigating the effects of oxidative stress and inflammation, both of which are major contributors to the aging process and the development of age-related diseases.

Furthermore, intermittent fasting has been linked to the activation of sirtuins, a class of proteins that regulate various cellular processes, including DNA repair, metabolism, and inflammation. By modulating the activity of these proteins, intermittent fasting may contribute to the maintenance of cellular health and potentially increase lifespan.

Research in animal models has also demonstrated the potential of intermittent fasting to extend lifespan and delay the onset of age-related diseases. While more human studies are needed to fully understand the implications for human longevity, the existing evidence suggests that implementing intermittent fasting as a lifestyle choice may align with the goal of optimizing vitality and promoting healthy aging.

# CHAPTER 3: GETTING STARTED WITH INTERMITTENT FASTING

Embarking on an intermittent fasting journey can be both exciting and daunting. The promise of sustainable weight loss and improved health is enticing, but knowing where to start is crucial. This chapter will provide you with practical guidance on initiating and maintaining an intermittent fasting routine, ensuring a smooth and successful transition.

## A Step-by-Step Guide to Starting Intermittent Fasting

Starting intermittent fasting doesn't have to be overwhelming. Begin by gradually increasing your fasting periods to allow your body to adapt to the new eating schedule. For instance, you might start with a 12-hour fast, from 7 PM to 7 AM, which includes your sleep time, making the transition easier. Over time, you can extend your fasting period to 14 and then 16 hours, finding a rhythm that suits your lifestyle.

Experimentation is key. There are various intermittent fasting methods, such as the 16/8 method, the 5:2 diet, and alternate-day fasting. The 16/8 method, where you fast for 16 hours and eat during an 8-hour window, is popular for its simplicity and effectiveness. Alternatively, the 5:2 diet involves eating normally for five days and restricting calories to 500-600 on two non-consecutive days. Find the method that aligns best with your daily routine and preferences.

Jennifer's journey with intermittent fasting began with a similar approach. She started with a 12-hour fast and gradually extended it to 16 hours. This gradual increase allowed her body to adapt without feeling deprived. Jennifer experimented with different methods and eventually settled on the 16/8 method, which fit seamlessly into her busy lifestyle as a mother and professional.

Keeping a journal can be incredibly helpful. Track your fasting hours, meals, and how you feel throughout the day. This practice allows you to identify patterns, such as increased energy levels and improved focus during fasting periods, which can motivate you to stick with the routine. Jennifer found that journaling helped her stay accountable and recognize the positive changes in her body and mind.

Hydration is crucial. Drink plenty of water, herbal teas, and black coffee during your fasting periods. When it's time to eat, focus on nutrient-dense foods like lean proteins, whole grains, fruits, and vegetables to ensure your body receives the necessary nutrients to thrive. Jennifer made sure to stay hydrated and chose wholesome foods during her eating windows, which supported her overall health and well-being.

Overcoming Common Challenges When Beginning Intermittent Fasting

Starting intermittent fasting can come with its challenges, but with the right strategies, you can overcome them. Initially, you might struggle with hunger pangs, especially in the morning. To ease into the fasting routine, gradually push your breakfast time later each day until you can comfortably skip it altogether. This gradual adjustment helps your body adapt without feeling deprived.

Incorporating healthy fats and protein-rich foods in your meals can keep you satiated and prevent overeating during your eating window. Foods like avocados, nuts, chicken, fish, and legumes are excellent choices that help you feel full and satisfied. Jennifer found that including these foods in her diet helped her manage hunger and maintain her fasting schedule.

Staying busy is another effective strategy. Schedule activities like walking, reading, or working on hobbies during your fasting hours to keep your mind off food and make the fasting period more manageable. Drinking herbal teas and black coffee can also help suppress your appetite and provide a sense of fullness. Jennifer often engaged in activities she enjoyed, such as gardening and reading, to distract herself from hunger during fasting periods.

## Setting Realistic Goals for Intermittent Fasting

Setting realistic goals is essential for long-term success with intermittent fasting. Focus on non-scale victories, such as increased energy, improved mental clarity, and better sleep quality. These positive changes can reinforce your commitment to intermittent fasting, even when the scale doesn't show immediate results.

Set specific and achievable goals, such as fasting for 16 hours daily, incorporating more vegetables into your meals, and exercising three times a week. These goals provide a clear path to follow and keep you motivated. Jennifer set similar goals, which helped her stay focused and track her progress.

Remember that intermittent fasting is a journey towards overall well-being. Practice patience, understanding that sustainable weight loss and health improvements take time. Celebrate small milestones, like completing your first week of intermittent fasting or noticing your clothes fitting better, to stay motivated and committed to your routine. Jennifer celebrated her milestones, which kept her motivated and positive throughout her journey.

## Creating a Personalized Intermittent Fasting Schedule

Creating a personalized intermittent fasting schedule is key to maintaining the practice long-term. Consider your daily routine, work schedule, and personal preferences when designing your fasting and eating windows. For example, if you prefer to have dinner with your family, you might choose a fasting window that allows you to eat from noon to 8 PM.

Experiment with different fasting durations and meal timings to find what works best for your body and lifestyle. Some people find the 16/8 method effective, while others might prefer the 5:2 diet or alternate-day fasting. Flexibility is important, so adjust your fasting routine as needed. Jennifer tailored her fasting schedule to fit her daily routine, which made it easier for her to stick to the plan.

Consistency is crucial. Maintain a regular fasting schedule to help your body adapt and optimize the benefits of intermittent fasting. Seek support from online communities or consult with a healthcare professional to tailor your intermittent fasting plan to your individual needs. This support can provide valuable insights and encouragement, helping you stay on track. Jennifer found support in online communities, which provided her with motivation and accountability.

By following these guidelines, you can embark on a sustainable and rewarding intermittent fasting journey, paving the way for lasting weight loss and improved health. Remember, the key to success is consistency, patience, and support. With the right mindset and tools, you can achieve your weight loss goals and transform your health.

Jennifer's story, introduced in the first chapter, serves as a testament to the transformative power of intermittent fasting. Her journey highlights the importance of finding a method that fits seamlessly into your lifestyle and the value of a supportive community. As you embark on your own intermittent fasting journey, keep Jennifer's experience in mind and remember that you, too, can achieve lasting change with the right approach.

# CHAPTER 4: INTERMITTENT FASTING FOR WEIGHT LOSS

Intermittent fasting has gained significant popularity as an effective strategy for weight loss, and for good reason. By strategically scheduling periods of fasting and eating, this approach can tap into the body's natural ability to burn fat for energy, leading to sustainable weight loss results. In this chapter, we will delve into the mechanisms behind how intermittent fasting promotes fat burning and explore strategies to maximize its effectiveness for achieving your desired body composition goals.

## Understanding the Role of Intermittent Fasting in Fat Burning and Weight Management

One of the primary draws of intermittent fasting is its ability to promote fat burning in a natural and sustainable manner. During fasting periods, the body enters a metabolic state where it is forced to tap into stored energy reserves, primarily in the form of fat. This process, known as fat oxidation, not only facilitates weight loss but also enhances overall metabolic health.

During fasting, the body experiences a cascade of hormonal changes that prime it for efficient fat burning. Insulin levels decrease, allowing the body to access and utilize stored fats more readily.

Additionally, intermittent fasting has been shown to increase the production of growth hormone and norepinephrine, both of which contribute to enhanced fat metabolism and preservation of lean muscle mass. Jennifer's journey with intermittent fasting began with a similar approach. She started with a 12-hour fast and gradually extended it to 16 hours. This gradual increase allowed her body to adapt without feeling deprived.

Jennifer experimented with different methods and eventually settled on the 16/8 method, which fit seamlessly into her busy lifestyle as a mother and professional. She found that the hormonal changes during fasting periods helped her body become more efficient at burning fat, leading to noticeable weight loss and improved energy levels.

## Strategies for Maximizing Weight Loss Results through Intermittent Fasting

While intermittent fasting is a powerful tool for weight loss, there are specific strategies that can further enhance its effectiveness and help you achieve your desired body composition goals.

- <u>Adjusting Fasting Durations and Meal Timings</u>: Experiment with different fasting durations and meal timings to find the approach that best aligns with your individual metabolic needs and lifestyle. Some individuals may thrive on a 16/8 protocol, while others may prefer alternate-day fasting or a modified approach.

- <u>Incorporating High-Intensity Interval Training (HIIT)</u>: Combining intermittent fasting with HIIT exercises during fasting periods can amplify fat-burning processes. HIIT workouts stimulate the release of catecholamines, hormones that promote the breakdown of stored fat for energy.

- <u>Monitoring Caloric Intake and Nutrient Density</u>: While intermittent fasting does not require strict calorie counting, it is essential to focus on nutrient-rich foods during your eating windows. Prioritize lean proteins, fiber-rich vegetables, and healthy fats to support satiety and maintain a calorie deficit conducive to weight loss.

- <u>Balancing Macronutrient Ratios</u>: Ensure adequate protein intake to preserve lean muscle mass while adjusting carbohydrate and fat ratios to align with your specific goals. A moderate-protein, low-carb approach during eating windows can further enhance fat-burning mechanisms.

- <u>Staying Hydrated and Replenishing Electrolytes</u>: Proper hydration and electrolyte balance are crucial during fasting periods to support overall health and prevent potential side effects like headaches or fatigue.

Jennifer found that incorporating these strategies into her routine made a significant difference. She combined her fasting schedule with regular HIIT workouts, which not only boosted her fat-burning potential but also improved her overall fitness. By focusing on nutrient-dense foods and staying hydrated, she was able to maintain her energy levels and avoid common pitfalls like fatigue and cravings.

## Targeting Stubborn Fat Areas with Intermittent Fasting

While intermittent fasting can promote overall fat loss, some individuals may struggle with stubborn fat deposits in specific areas, such as the abdomen or thighs. In these cases, a strategic approach can help target these stubborn fat regions more effectively.

- <u>Reducing Visceral Fat</u>: Intermittent fasting has been shown to be particularly effective in reducing visceral fat, the dangerous fat that accumulates around the abdominal organs. By lowering insulin levels and promoting fat oxidation, intermittent fasting can help shrink waistlines and improve overall metabolic health.

- <u>Combining Fasting with Targeted Strength Training</u>: Incorporating strength training exercises that target specific muscle groups can help tone and sculpt areas prone to stubborn fat accumulation. As you build muscle in these areas, your body's metabolic rate will increase, further supporting fat loss.

- <u>Enhancing Blood Flow</u>: Stubborn fat areas often

- have poor blood flow, which can hinder the delivery of fat-burning hormones to these regions. Strategies like intermittent fasting, low-carb diets, and the use of compression garments like the Shred Belt can help increase blood flow, facilitating the mobilization of stubborn fat deposits.

- <u>Maintaining Moderate Physical Activity</u>: While intense exercise during fasting periods may not be advisable for everyone, engaging in moderate physical activity can help keep your blood flowing and prevent the re-deposition of mobilized fat into stubborn areas.

Jennifer noticed that her abdominal fat was particularly resistant to change. By incorporating targeted strength training exercises and using compression garments, she was able to enhance blood flow to this area and see more significant results. Her persistence and strategic approach paid off, leading to a more toned and sculpted physique.

## Preserving Muscle Mass During Weight Loss with Intermittent Fasting

One of the significant advantages of intermittent fasting is its ability to promote weight loss while preserving lean muscle mass. However, to fully capitalize on this benefit, it is essential to incorporate specific strategies into your routine.

- <u>Prioritizing Protein Intake</u>: Consuming an adequate amount of high-quality protein within your eating windows is crucial for preserving and building muscle mass. Aim for a protein intake of 0.5-0.8 grams per pound of body weight, depending on your activity level and goals.

- <u>Incorporating Resistance Training</u>: Combining intermittent fasting with a structured resistance training program can help maintain and even build lean muscle mass. Resistance exercises stimulate muscle protein synthesis, counteracting the potential for muscle loss during fasting periods.

- <u>Ensuring Proper Recovery</u>: Adequate rest and sleep are essential for muscle repair and growth. Prioritize quality sleep and allow for sufficient recovery between resistance training sessions to support muscle preservation and development.

- <u>Monitoring Body Composition Changes</u>: Regularly assessing your body composition, beyond just weight measurements, can provide valuable insights into your progress. Track changes in body fat percentage and lean muscle mass to make informed adjustments to your fasting regimen and exercise routine.

By following these strategies, you can effectively leverage the power of intermittent fasting for sustainable weight loss while maintaining a lean, toned physique and optimizing your overall body.

# CHAPTER 5: MEAL PLANNING AND RECIPES FOR INTERMITTENT FASTING

One of the keys to success is having a well-structured meal plan that ensures you get the necessary nutrients while adhering to your fasting schedule. In this chapter, we will guide you through the essentials of meal planning and provide a variety of nutritious recipes to help you make the most of your intermittent fasting routine.

## The Importance of Meal Planning

Effective meal planning is crucial for anyone practicing intermittent fasting. It ensures that you have nutritious meals ready, preventing impulsive food choices during eating windows. By planning your meals in advance, you can maintain a balanced diet, ensuring adequate intake of essential nutrients within your fasting periods. This approach not only aids in weight management but also supports overall health and well-being.

Jennifer found that meal planning was a game-changer in her intermittent fasting journey. By dedicating time each week to plan her meals, she was able to avoid the pitfalls of unhealthy snacking and ensure she was consuming nutrient-dense foods. This preparation helped her stay on track and made her fasting periods more manageable.

# Creating Balanced and Satisfying Meals

When planning your meals, it's important to incorporate a variety of nutrient-dense foods. Focus on lean proteins, whole grains, fruits, and vegetables to ensure a well-rounded meal that satisfies hunger and provides essential nutrients. Experiment with different meal combinations to keep your intermittent fasting meals interesting and enjoyable. Utilize herbs, spices, and healthy fats to enhance the flavor of your meals without adding unnecessary calories.

Jennifer enjoyed experimenting with different recipes and found that incorporating a variety of flavors and textures made her meals more satisfying. She often prepared dishes like grilled chicken with quinoa and roasted vegetables, or a hearty lentil soup with a side of fresh salad. These meals not only kept her full but also provided the nutrients her body needed to thrive.

## Sample Meal Plan for Intermittent Fasting

To help you get started, here is a sample meal plan for a full day of intermittent fasting, with balanced and nutritious meals within the eating window. Remember to stay hydrated with water, herbal teas, or black coffee during fasting hours.

<u>Breakfast (12:00 PM): Green Smoothie</u>
- 1 avocado
- 1 cup coconut milk

- 1 small handful blueberries
- 1 cup spinach, kale, or chard
- 1 tablespoon chia seeds

Lunch (3:00 PM): Grilled Chicken Salad

- 1 grilled chicken breast
- Mixed greens (spinach, arugula, kale)
- Cherry tomatoes, cucumber, and bell peppers
- 1 tablespoon olive oil and lemon juice dressing

Snack (5:00 PM): Greek Yogurt with Berries

- 1 cup Greek yogurt
- 1/2 cup mixed berries (blueberries, strawberries, raspberries)
- 1 tablespoon honey

Dinner (7:00 PM): Baked Salmon with Quinoa and Steamed Vegetables

- 1 salmon fillet
- 1 cup cooked quinoa
- Steamed broccoli, carrots, and zucchini
- 1 tablespoon olive oil

These are just a few recipes to get you started. At the end of this book, you will find 35 additional bonus recipes designed to fit seamlessly into your intermittent fasting plan, ensuring you have plenty of delicious and nutritious options to choose from.

## Practical Tips for Meal Prepping and Batch Cooking

Meal prepping and batch cooking can streamline your intermittent fasting routine, making it easier to stick to your fasting plan and resist the temptation to break your fast with unhealthy choices. Dedicate a specific day for meal prepping, where you can cook in bulk and store individual portions for the week. Invest in quality storage containers and labels to organize your prepped meals and snacks for easy access and portion control.

Jennifer found that setting aside time on Sundays to prepare her meals for the week was incredibly helpful. She would cook large batches of quinoa, grill several chicken breasts, and chop a variety of vegetables. This preparation allowed her to quickly assemble meals during her eating windows, saving time and reducing stress.

By planning your meals in advance and incorporating a range of nutrient-dense foods, you can ensure that you stay on track and make the most of your fasting periods. With these tools and recipes, you are well-equipped to embark on a sustainable and enjoyable intermittent fasting journey.

# CHAPTER 6: ACCELERATING FAT LOSS WITH ADVANCED INTERMITTENT FASTING

As you progress on your intermittent fasting journey, you may find yourself hitting a plateau or seeking ways to accelerate your fat loss. Advanced intermittent fasting techniques can help you break through these barriers and achieve your weight loss goals more efficiently. In this chapter, we will explore various advanced strategies to enhance fat burning and optimize your intermittent fasting routine.

## Incorporating Longer Fasting Periods

One effective way to boost fat loss is by incorporating longer fasting periods into your routine. Extending your fasting window can enhance fat oxidation and increase your metabolic rate, leading to greater weight loss outcomes. For example, transitioning from a 16/8 fasting schedule to an 18/6 or even a 20/4 schedule can provide your body with more time to burn stored fat for energy.

Jennifer experienced significant benefits when she extended her fasting periods. Initially, she followed a 16/8 schedule, but as she became more comfortable with fasting, she experimented with an 18/6 schedule. This adjustment allowed her body to tap into fat stores more effectively, resulting in accelerated fat loss and improved energy levels.

## Exploring Alternate-Day Fasting

Alternate-day fasting (ADF) is another advanced technique that can help you overcome weight loss plateaus. This method involves alternating between days of regular eating and fasting. On fasting days, you consume very few calories (about 500-600), while on non-fasting days, you eat normally. This approach promotes calorie restriction without long-term deprivation, making it a sustainable option for many people.

Research has shown that alternate-day fasting can lead to significant weight loss and improvements in metabolic health. By reducing overall caloric intake and enhancing insulin sensitivity, ADF can support sustainable weight management. Jennifer found that incorporating ADF into her routine helped her break through a weight loss plateau and continue making progress towards her goals.

## Breaking Weight Loss Plateaus with Advanced Techniques

Hitting a weight loss plateau can be frustrating, but advanced intermittent fasting techniques can help you overcome this challenge. One strategy is to increase the duration of your fasting periods or modify your fasting protocols. For example, you might try a 24-hour fast once a week or incorporate a fasting-mimicking diet for a few days.

Jennifer faced a plateau after several months of intermittent fasting. To break through it, she experimented with a 24-hour fast once a week. This change helped her body reset and jumpstart her fat-burning processes, allowing her to continue losing weight.

Another effective approach is to incorporate strategic meal timing and composition changes. For instance, focusing on nutrient-dense, low-carb meals during your eating windows can enhance fat-burning mechanisms. Additionally, incorporating high-intensity interval training (HIIT) during fasting periods can boost your metabolism and accelerate fat loss.

## Maintaining Muscle Mass During Advanced Fasting

One of the significant advantages of intermittent fasting is its ability to promote weight loss while preserving lean muscle mass. However, as you incorporate advanced fasting techniques, it's essential to prioritize muscle maintenance to ensure a balanced and healthy body composition.

- <u>Prioritizing Protein Intake</u>: Consuming an adequate amount of high-quality protein within your eating windows is crucial for preserving and building muscle mass. Aim for a protein intake of 0.5-0.8 grams per pound of body weight, depending on your activity level and goals.

- <u>Incorporating Resistance Training</u>: Combining intermittent fasting with a structured resistance training program can help maintain and even build lean muscle mass. Resistance exercises stimulate muscle protein synthesis, counteracting the potential for muscle loss during fasting periods.

- <u>Ensuring Proper Recovery</u>: Adequate rest and sleep are essential for muscle repair and growth. Prioritize quality sleep and allow for sufficient recovery between resistance training sessions to support muscle preservation and development.

- <u>Monitoring Body Composition Changes</u>: Regularly assessing your body composition, beyond just weight measurements, can provide valuable insights into your progress. Track changes in body fat percentage and lean muscle mass to make informed adjustments to your fasting regimen and exercise routine.

By incorporating longer fasting periods, exploring alternate-day fasting, and making strategic adjustments to your fasting protocols, you can enhance your fat-burning potential and achieve your weight loss goals more efficiently.

# CHAPTER 7: INTERMITTENT FASTING AND EXERCISE

Combining intermittent fasting with regular physical activity can amplify the benefits and accelerate your journey towards achieving your desired body transformation. In this chapter, we will explore the synergistic relationship between intermittent fasting and exercise, providing you with practical strategies to optimize your workouts and support your overall fitness goals.

## The Benefits of Combining Intermittent Fasting and Exercise

Intermittent fasting and exercise are powerful allies in the pursuit of weight loss and improved overall health. When combined effectively, they can create a potent synergy that enhances fat-burning mechanisms and supports the preservation of lean muscle mass.

One of the primary advantages of exercising during fasting periods is the body's increased ability to tap into stored fat reserves for energy. As insulin levels decrease during fasting, the body becomes more efficient at utilizing fat as fuel, a process known as fat oxidation. This metabolic state can be further amplified by engaging in physical activity, leading to accelerated fat loss.

Additionally, intermittent fasting has been shown to boost the production of growth hormone and norepinephrine, hormones that play a crucial role in promoting fat metabolism and preserving lean muscle mass. By incorporating exercise into your intermittent fasting routine, you can maximize the benefits of these hormonal changes, supporting your body composition goals.

## Choosing the Right Workouts for Intermittent Fasting

When it comes to exercising during intermittent fasting, it's essential to select workouts that align with your energy levels and personal preferences. Here are some effective options to consider:

- <u>High-Intensity Interval Training (HIIT)</u>: HIIT workouts, which involve short bursts of intense exercise followed by periods of rest or lower-intensity activity, are particularly effective during fasting periods. These workouts stimulate the release of catecholamines, hormones that promote the breakdown of stored fat for energy.

- <u>Low-Impact Activities</u>: If you find yourself feeling fatigued during fasting periods, low-impact activities like yoga, Pilates, or light walking can be excellent choices. These exercises can enhance flexibility, reduce stress, and promote overall well-being without overly taxing your body.

- <u>Endurance Exercises</u>: Activities like jogging, cycling, or swimming can be sustained well in a fasted state, as the body becomes more efficient at utilizing fat for fuel during these exercises.

Remember, it's crucial to listen to your body's cues and adjust the intensity of your workouts based on your energy levels while fasting. If you feel dizzy, lightheaded, or excessively fatigued, it's best to take a break or opt for a lower-intensity activity.

## Fueling Your Workouts During Intermittent Fasting

While exercising in a fasted state can be beneficial, it's essential to ensure proper hydration and nutrient intake to support your performance and recovery. Here are some tips for fueling your workouts during intermittent fasting:

- <u>Stay Hydrated</u>: Drink plenty of water and electrolyte-rich beverages like coconut water or sports drinks (without added sugars) to replenish fluids lost during exercise and prevent dehydration.

- <u>Pre-Workout Snacks</u>: If you find it challenging to exercise on an empty stomach, consider having a small, nutrient-dense snack like a handful of nuts or a piece of fruit before your workout. This can provide a quick energy boost without disrupting your fasting period significantly.

- <u>Post-Workout Meals</u>: After your workout, break your fast with a balanced meal that includes a combination of protein, complex carbohydrates, and healthy fats. This will help replenish your energy stores, support muscle recovery, and promote overall nutrient balance.

- <u>Experiment and Adjust</u>: Everyone's body responds differently to exercise during fasting periods. Experiment with different timing and compositions of pre- and post-workout meals to find what works best for your body and supports your performance and recovery.

## Example Workout Plan with Jennifer

Jennifer's journey with intermittent fasting and exercise provides a practical example of how to integrate these two powerful strategies effectively. Here is a sample weekly workout plan that Jennifer followed, combining intermittent fasting with various types of exercise:

<u>Monday:</u>

- Morning: Fasted cardio (30 minutes of brisk walking)
- 12 PM: Break fast with a protein-rich meal (e.g., scrambled eggs with spinach and avocado)
- Afternoon: Light stretching or yoga

<u>Tuesday</u>:

- Morning: Strength training (focus on upper body)
- 12 PM: Break fast with a balanced meal (e.g., grilled chicken salad with mixed greens and quinoa)
- Evening: Light walk or gentle Pilates

<u>Wednesday</u>:

- Morning: Fasted HIIT workout (20 minutes of high-intensity intervals)
- 12 PM: Break fast with a nutrient-dense meal (e.g., smoothie with protein powder, berries, and almond milk)
- Afternoon: Rest or light stretching

<u>Thursday</u>:

- Morning: Endurance exercise (45 minutes of cycling)
- 12 PM: Break fast with a balanced meal (e.g., salmon with sweet potatoes and steamed vegetables)
- Evening: Light walk or restorative yoga

<u>Friday</u>:

- Morning: Strength training (focus on lower body)
- 12 PM: Break fast with a protein-rich meal (e.g., turkey and vegetable stir-fry with brown rice)
- Evening: Light stretching or yoga

<u>Saturday:</u>

- Morning: Fasted cardio (30 minutes of jogging)
- 12 PM: Break fast with a balanced meal (e.g., Greek yogurt with mixed berries and nuts)
- Afternoon: Light walk or gentle Pilates

<u>Sunday:</u>

- Rest Day: Focus on hydration, light stretching, and self-care activities

## Maintaining Energy Levels and Performance

Exercising while intermittent fasting can be challenging, especially during the initial adjustment period. To maintain optimal energy levels and performance, consider the following strategies:

- <u>Listen to Your Body's Hunger Cues</u>: Pay attention to your body's signals and adjust the timing of your workouts accordingly. If you feel excessively hungry or fatigued, it may be best to schedule your exercise session closer to your eating window.

- <u>Monitor Fatigue and Dizziness</u>: Stay mindful of any signs of excessive fatigue or dizziness during your workouts. If you experience these symptoms, take breaks or adjust the intensity levels as needed to prioritize your safety and well-being.

- <u>Establish a Consistent Routine</u>: As your body adapts to the combination of intermittent fasting and exercise, establish a consistent workout routine within your fasting periods. This consistency will help your body become more efficient at utilizing stored energy reserves, improving your energy levels over time.

- <u>Prioritize Rest and Recovery</u>: Adequate rest and recovery are crucial for muscle repair and preventing burnout. Ensure you get enough sleep and allow for sufficient recovery time between intense workout sessions to support your body's recovery processes.

Combining intermittent fasting with regular exercise can be a powerful strategy for achieving your desired body transformation. By understanding the synergistic relationship between these two practices and implementing the strategies outlined in this chapter, you can maximize fat-burning potential, preserve lean muscle mass, and support overall health and well-being. Remember to listen to your body, stay hydrated, and prioritize proper nutrition and recovery to ensure a safe and effective journey towards your fitness goals.

# CHAPTER 8: ADDRESSING COMMON MISCONCEPTIONS ABOUT INTERMITTENT FASTING

Intermittent fasting has gained significant popularity, but with its rise, several myths and misconceptions have also emerged. These myths can deter people from trying intermittent fasting or lead to misunderstandings about its effects. In this chapter, we will debunk some of the most common myths about intermittent fasting and provide evidence-based insights to help you make informed decisions.

## Myth 1: Intermittent Fasting Slows Down Your Metabolism

One of the most pervasive myths about intermittent fasting is that it puts your body into "starvation mode," slowing down your metabolism and preventing fat loss. This misconception stems from the idea that prolonged calorie restriction can lead to metabolic slowdown.

The Truth:

Intermittent fasting, when done correctly, does not slow down your metabolism. In fact, short-term fasting can boost metabolic function. During fasting periods, the body undergoes a metabolic shift from burning glycogen (carbohydrates and sugar) to using stored fat for fuel. This shift increases norepinephrine levels, a hormone that stimulates metabolism and accelerates fat breakdown. Studies have shown that intermittent fasting can enhance metabolic health and improve insulin sensitivity, which supports weight loss and overall metabolic function.

## Myth 2: Intermittent Fasting Causes Muscle Loss

Another common concern is that intermittent fasting leads to muscle loss. This myth is based on the belief that reducing meal frequency limits the body's ability to support muscle development.

The Truth:

Intermittent fasting does not inherently cause muscle loss if you maintain adequate protein intake and engage in regular resistance training. Fasting periods can actually increase the production of growth hormones, which are essential for muscle preservation and growth. Research indicates that intermittent fasting can be more effective at preserving lean muscle mass compared to continuous calorie restriction diets. To prevent muscle loss, focus on consuming protein-rich meals during your eating windows and incorporate strength training exercises into your routine.

## Myth 3: Intermittent Fasting Causes Nutrient Deficiencies

Some people worry that intermittent fasting leads to nutrient deficiencies due to reduced calorie intake and limited eating windows.

The Truth:

Intermittent fasting can improve nutrient absorption and digestive efficiency by giving your digestive system valuable periods of rest. However, like any dietary pattern, it is crucial to plan your meals properly to ensure you consume a variety of nutrient-dense foods. Nutrient deficiencies are more likely to occur if you do not follow a balanced diet or if you implement extreme fasting methods, such as fasting for more than 24 hours without proper nutrition. Focus on eating whole foods, including fruits, vegetables, lean proteins, and healthy fats, to meet your nutritional needs.

## Myth 4: Intermittent Fasting is Unsafe

There is a misconception that intermittent fasting is inherently unsafe and can lead to health issues such as dehydration, malnutrition, or metabolic imbalances.

The Truth:

Intermittent fasting is generally safe for most healthy individuals when done correctly. It is important to stay hydrated and consume nutrient-dense foods during eating windows to avoid potential side effects like headaches, lethargy, or constipation. However, certain groups of people, such as those with a history of eating disorders, pregnant or breastfeeding women, and individuals with specific medical conditions, should consult a healthcare professional before starting intermittent fasting. As with any dietary change, it is essential to listen to your body and make adjustments as needed.

## Myth 5: You Can Eat Anything You Want During Eating Windows

Some people believe that intermittent fasting allows you to eat anything you want during your eating windows without considering the quality of the food.

The Truth:

While intermittent fasting focuses on when you eat rather than what you eat, the quality of your food still matters. Consuming nutrient-dense foods is crucial for overall health and weight management. Overeating unhealthy foods during eating windows can negate the benefits of fasting and lead to weight gain. Aim for a balanced diet that includes whole grains, lean proteins, healthy fats, fruits, and vegetables to support your health and fasting goals.

## Myth 6: Intermittent Fasting is a Miracle Cure for Weight Loss

Intermittent fasting is often touted as a miracle solution for weight loss, leading some to believe that it guarantees rapid and effortless results.

The Truth:

Intermittent fasting can be an effective tool for weight loss, but it is not a miracle cure. Sustainable weight loss requires a combination of healthy eating, regular physical activity, and a balanced lifestyle. Intermittent fasting helps create a calorie deficit and improve metabolic health, but it should be part of a comprehensive approach to weight management. Setting realistic goals and maintaining consistency are key to achieving long-term success.

## Myth 7: Intermittent Fasting is Suitable for Everyone

There is a belief that intermittent fasting is a one-size-fits-all solution that works for everyone.

The Truth:

Intermittent fasting is not suitable for everyone. Individual responses to fasting can vary based on factors such as age, gender, health status, and lifestyle. Some people may thrive on intermittent fasting, while others may find it challenging or unsuitable for their needs. It is important to find a dietary approach that aligns with your personal preferences and health goals. Consulting with a healthcare professional can help determine if intermittent fasting is right for you.

# CHAPTER 9: EMBRACING A SUSTAINABLE LIFESTYLE WITH INTERMITTENT FASTING

Intermittent fasting is more than just a diet; it's a lifestyle that can be seamlessly integrated into your daily routine for long-term health benefits. This chapter will guide you on how to make intermittent fasting a sustainable part of your life, ensuring that you can maintain your progress and enjoy the benefits for years to come.

## Integrating Intermittent Fasting into Daily Routines

One of the keys to making intermittent fasting sustainable is to integrate it into your daily routine in a way that feels natural and manageable. Start by identifying optimal fasting and eating windows that align with your daily schedule. For instance, if you have a traditional 9-5 job, you might find it easier to skip breakfast and have your eating window from 12 PM to 8 PM. This way, you can enjoy lunch and dinner without feeling rushed or deprived.

Jennifer found that planning her fasting schedule around her work and family commitments made it easier to stick to her routine. She would often prepare her meals in advance, ensuring she had nutritious options ready when her eating window opened. This preparation helped her avoid impulsive eating and stay on track with her fasting goals.

## Staying Consistent and Motivated

Consistency is crucial for long-term success with intermittent fasting. Establishing a support system can provide the accountability and encouragement needed to stay motivated. Join online communities or find a fasting buddy who shares your goals. Sharing your experiences and challenges with others can provide valuable insights and keep you motivated.

Setting short-term goals and celebrating milestones can also boost motivation. Jennifer set weekly goals, such as fasting for a certain number of hours or incorporating more vegetables into her meals. Celebrating these small victories helped her stay focused and committed to her long-term goals.

Practicing mindfulness and self-awareness around eating habits can enhance self-control and discipline. Jennifer found that engaging in enjoyable activities during fasting periods, such as reading or taking a walk, helped distract her from hunger and made the experience more positive.

## Transitioning from Weight Loss to Weight Maintenance

Once you achieve your weight loss goals, transitioning to a maintenance phase is essential to sustain your progress. Gradually adjust your fasting schedule to include maintenance calories while still reaping the metabolic benefits of intermittent fasting. This might mean slightly shortening your fasting window or incorporating occasional refeed days.

Emphasize nutrient-dense foods and mindful eating practices to support weight maintenance and overall health. Incorporate regular physical activity and stay hydrated to enhance vitality and prevent weight regain. Monitoring your progress and making adjustments based on your needs and goals will help you maintain your achievements over time.

Jennifer successfully transitioned to a maintenance phase by gradually increasing her calorie intake and continuing her fasting routine. She focused on balanced meals and regular exercise, which helped her maintain her weight and overall well-being.

## Psychological Benefits of Intermittent Fasting

Intermittent fasting offers numerous psychological benefits beyond physical health. Many people report increased mental clarity and focus during fasting periods. This mental sharpness can enhance productivity and cognitive function, making it easier to tackle daily tasks.
Fasting also cultivates discipline and resilience, which

can translate into other areas of life. Jennifer found that the self-control she developed through fasting helped her make healthier choices in other aspects of her life, such as managing stress and prioritizing self-care.

Addressing emotional connections to food and practicing mindful eating can foster a healthier relationship with food. By focusing on how foods make you feel rather than labeling them as "good" or "bad," you can develop a more balanced and positive mindset.

Prioritizing self-care practices like stress management and adequate sleep alongside intermittent fasting can enhance mental and emotional resilience. Jennifer made it a point to get enough rest and engage in activities that brought her joy, which supported her overall well-being.

Embracing intermittent fasting as a sustainable lifestyle choice involves integrating it into your daily routine, staying consistent and motivated, transitioning to weight maintenance, and enjoying the psychological benefits. By finding a balance that works for you and prioritizing holistic wellness practices, you can make intermittent fasting a long-term part of your life.

# CHAPTER 10: PERSONALIZING YOUR INTERMITTENT FASTING JOURNEY

Intermittent fasting is a versatile and adaptable approach to health and weight management, but its success largely depends on how well it fits into your individual lifestyle and preferences. This chapter will guide you on how to personalize your intermittent fasting journey, ensuring it aligns with your unique needs and goals.

## Assessing Lifestyle Factors

The first step in personalizing your intermittent fasting plan is to assess your lifestyle factors. Consider your work schedule, social commitments, exercise routine, and personal preferences. Understanding these elements will help you choose a fasting plan that is sustainable and enjoyable.

Jennifer, a busy mother of two with a demanding job, found that the 16/8 method worked best for her. She skipped breakfast and had her eating window from 12 PM to 8 PM, which allowed her to have lunch and dinner with her family. This schedule fit seamlessly into her daily routine and helped her stay consistent with her fasting goals.

## Personalizing Fasting Windows

aTiloring your fasting and eating periods to align with your daily habits is crucial for long-term adherence. Experiment with different fasting windows to find what works best for you. Some people prefer the 16/8 method, while others might find the 18/6 or 20/4 schedules more effective.

Tips for Personalization:

- <u>Morning Person</u>: If you are more active in the morning, consider an eating window that starts earlier in the day, such as 8 AM to 4 PM.

- <u>Night Owl</u>: If you prefer late-night activities, an eating window from 2 PM to 10 PM might be more suitable.

- <u>Flexible Schedule</u>: If your daily routine varies, consider a more flexible approach like the 5:2 diet, where you fast for two non-consecutive days each week.

## Incorporating Flexibility

Flexibility is key to maintaining a sustainable intermittent fasting routine. Life is unpredictable, and there will be days when sticking to your fasting schedule is challenging. Allow yourself the flexibility to adjust your fasting periods based on your circumstances.

Jennifer occasionally had social events or family gatherings that fell outside her usual eating window. Instead of feeling guilty or stressed, she adjusted her fasting schedule for those days, ensuring she could enjoy the event without compromising her overall progress.

## Seeking Professional Guidance

If you have specific health conditions or dietary needs, consulting with a healthcare provider or nutrition expert can help you customize your intermittent fasting plan safely and effectively. Professional guidance can provide personalized recommendations and address any concerns you may have.

## Exploring Different Eating Patterns

Intermittent fasting can be adapted to various dietary preferences and restrictions. Whether you follow a vegan, keto, or gluten-free diet, you can tailor your fasting plan to suit your needs.

Tips for Adaptation:

- <u>Vegan</u>: Focus on plant-based proteins like legumes, tofu, and quinoa during your eating windows.

- <u>Keto</u>: Incorporate high-fat, low-carb foods such as avocados, nuts, and fatty fish.

- <u>Gluten-Free</u>: Choose gluten-free grains like rice, quinoa, and gluten-free oats.

## Monitoring Progress and Making Adjustments

Tracking your progress is crucial for optimizing your intermittent fasting journey. Use apps or journals to record your fasting durations, meal choices, and energy levels. Regularly assess your physical responses and make necessary adjustments to your fasting protocols.

Jennifer used a fasting app to log her fasting hours and meals. She also noted her energy levels and mood, which helped her identify patterns and make informed changes to her routine.

Personalizing your intermittent fasting journey involves understanding your lifestyle, experimenting with different fasting windows, and making adjustments based on your needs and preferences. By incorporating flexibility, seeking professional guidance, and building sustainable habits, you can create a fasting routine that aligns with your goals and enhances your overall health.

# CHAPTER 11: YOUR 28 DAY WEIGHT LOSS TRANSFORMATION

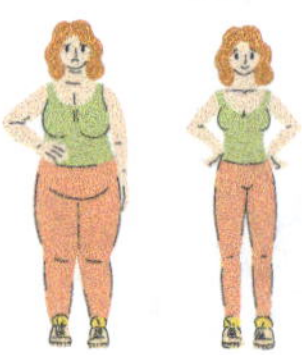

This 28-day intermittent fasting plan is designed to help you lose weight progressively, starting with easier fasting schedules and gradually moving to more advanced methods. By the end of this plan, you can expect to lose approximately 8-12 pounds, depending on your starting point, adherence to the guidelines, and individual metabolic rate.

## TIPS FOR MAINTAINING PROGRESS BEYOND 28 DAYS

1. <u>Gradual Transition</u>: After completing the 28-day plan, gradually adjust your fasting schedule to include maintenance calories while still reaping the metabolic benefits of intermittent fasting.

2. <u>Balanced Nutrition</u>: Continue to focus on nutrient-dense foods and mindful eating practices to support weight maintenance and overall health.

3. <u>Regular Exercise</u>: Incorporate regular physical activity into your routine to enhance vitality and prevent weight regain.

4. <u>Hydration and Sleep</u>: Prioritize hydration and adequate sleep to support your body's rejuvenation processes.

5. <u>Monitor Progress</u>: Regularly assess your progress and make adjustments based on your needs and goals to sustain your weight loss results.

# WEEK 1: INTRODUCTION TO INTERMITTENT FASTING

## FASTING SCHEDULE

Fasting Period: 12 hours
(8 PM to 8 AM)

Eating Window: 12 hours
(8 AM to 8 PM)

## MEAL PLAN

Breakfast (8 AM)

Lunch (12 PM)

Snack (3 PM)

Dinner (7 PM)

## NOTES

**MONDAY**

30 minutes of brisk walking or light jogging

**TUESDAY**

20 minutes of yoga or stretching exercises

**WEDNESDAY**

30 minutes of brisk walking or light jogging

**THURSDAY**

20 minutes of yoga or stretching exercises

**FRIDAY**

30 minutes of brisk walking or light jogging

**WEEKEND**

Saturday: Rest day
Sunday: 30 minutes of light cardio (e.g. cycling or swimming)

# WEEK 2: INCREASING THE CHALLENGE

## FASTING SCHEDULE

Fasting Period: 14 hours (8 PM to 10 AM)

Eating Window: 10 hours (10 AM to 8 PM)

## MEAL PLAN

Breakfast (10 AM)

Lunch (1 PM)

Snack (4 PM)

Dinner (7 PM)

## NOTES

**MONDAY**

10 minutes of HIIT (High-Intensity Interval Training)

**TUESDAY**

20 minutes of Pilates or core exercises

**WEDNESDAY**

10 minutes of HIIT (High-Intensity Interval Training)

**THURSDAY**

20 minutes of Pilates or core exercises

**FRIDAY**

10 minutes of HIIT (High-Intensity Interval Training)

**WEEKEND**

Saturday: Rest day
Sunday: 30 minutes of moderate cardio (e.g. brisk walking or cycling)

# WEEK 3: ADVANCING FURTHER

## FASTING SCHEDULE

Fasting Period: 16 hours (8 PM to 12 PM)

Eating Window: 8 hours (12 PM to 8 PM)

## MEAL PLAN

Breakfast (12 PM)

Lunch (3 PM)

Snack (5 PM)

Dinner (7 PM)

## NOTES

### MONDAY

40 minutes of strength training (focus on different muscle groups each day)

### TUESDAY

30 minutes of HIIT

### WEDNESDAY

40 minutes of strength training (focus on different muscle groups each day)

### THURSDAY

30 minutes of HIIT

### FRIDAY

40 minutes of strength training (focus on different muscle groups each day)

### WEEKEND

Saturday: Rest day
Sunday: 30 minutes of light cardio and stretching

# WEEK 4: OPTIMIZING AND THRIVING

## FASTING SCHEDULE

Fasting Period: 16 hours
(8 PM to 12 PM)

Eating Window: 8 hours
(12 PM to 8 PM)

## MEAL PLAN

Breakfast (2 PM)

Snack (4 PM)

Dinner (7 PM)

## NOTES

### MONDAY

45 minutes of strength training and 15 minutes of cardio

### TUESDAY

30 minutes of HIIT and 15 minutes of core exercises

### WEDNESDAY

45 minutes of strength training and 15 minutes of cardio

### THURSDAY

30 minutes of HIIT and 15 minutes of core exercises

### FRIDAY

45 minutes of strength training and 15 minutes of cardio)

### WEEKEND

Saturday: Rest day
Sunday: 30 minutes of yoga or stretching

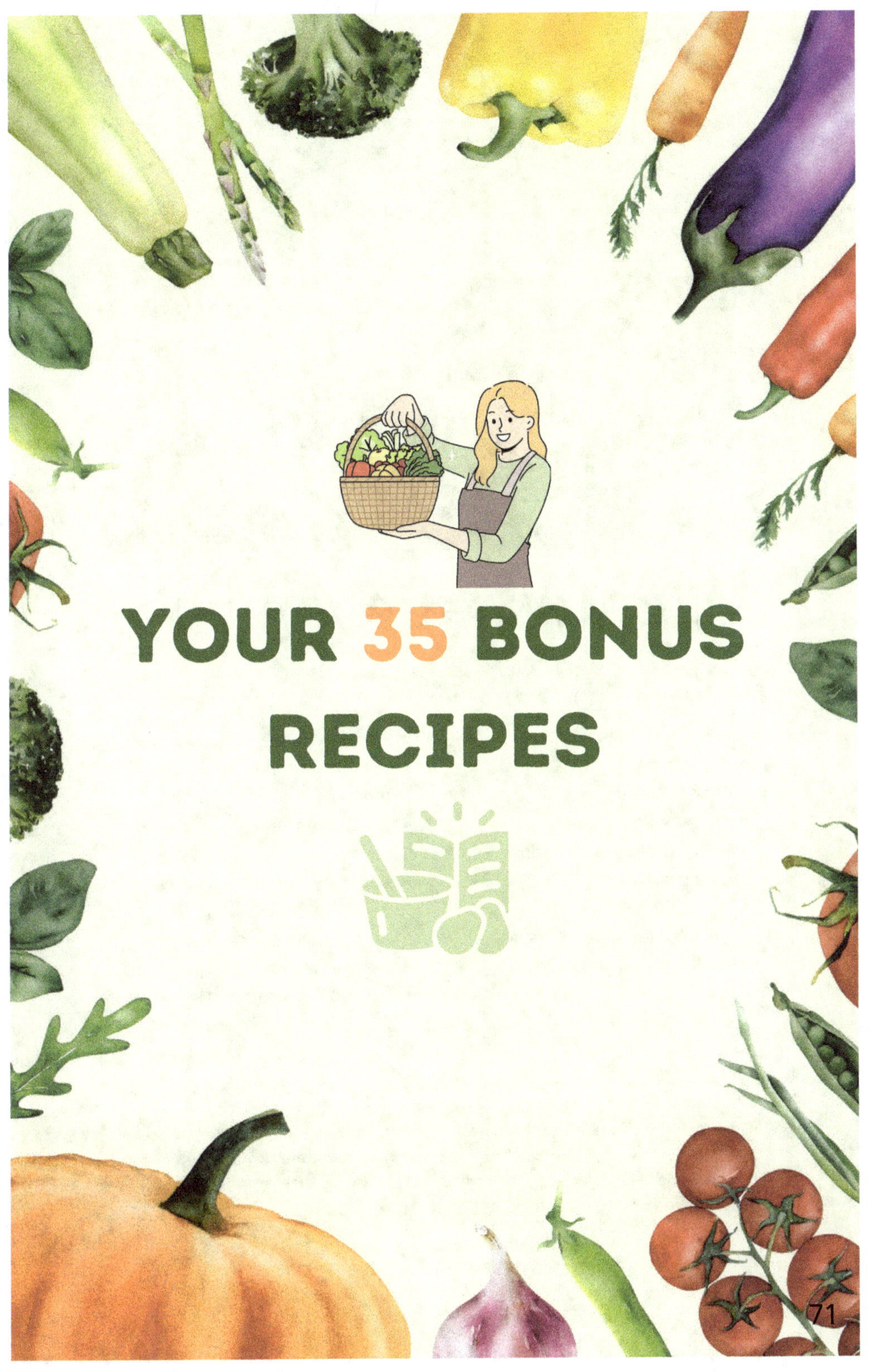

# YOUR 35 BONUS RECIPES

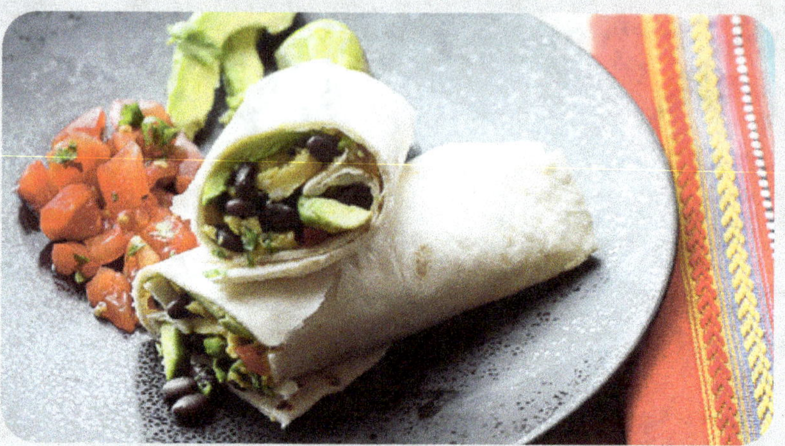

# BREAKFAST BURRITO

## Ingredients:

- 1 wholemeal wrap
- 2 eggs, scrambled
- 1/2 avocado, sliced
- 1/4 cup black beans, rinsed and drained
- 1/4 cup diced tomatoes
- 1/4 cup shredded cheese
- Salt and pepper to taste

## Instructions:

- Heat the wrap in a skillet over medium heat until warm.
- Scramble the eggs in a separate pan.
- Layer the scrambled eggs, avocado, black beans, tomatoes, and cheese on the wrap.
- Season with salt and pepper.
- Roll up the wrap and serve immediately.

Packed with protein and fiber, breakfast burritos provide lasting energy to power you through the morning. The combination of eggs, beans, and veggies makes it a nutrient-dense meal that supports muscle repair and digestive health.

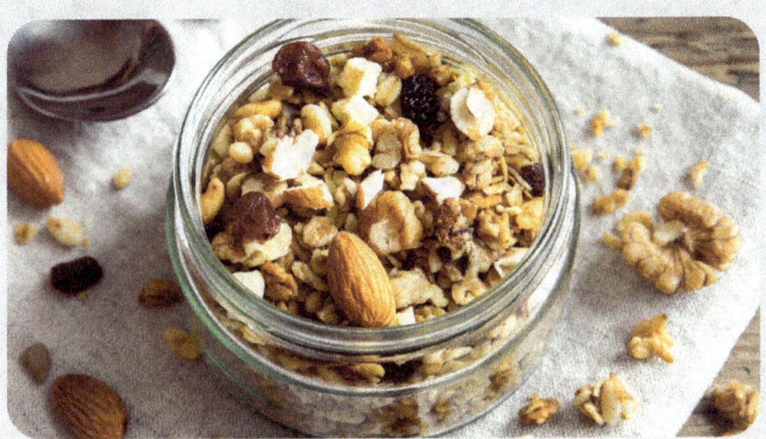

# HEALTHY HOMEMADE GRANOLA

## Ingredients:

- 2 cups rolled oats
- 1/2 cup chopped nuts (almonds, walnuts, or pecans)
- 1/4 cup honey or maple syrup
- 1/4 cup coconut oil, melted
- 1/2 cup dried fruit (raisins, cranberries, or apricots)
- 1 tsp vanilla extract
- 1/2 tsp cinnamon

## Instructions:

- Preheat the oven to 300°F (150°C).
- In a large bowl, mix the oats, nuts, honey, coconut oil, vanilla extract, and cinnamon.
- Spread the mixture evenly on a baking sheet lined with parchment paper.
- Bake for 20-25 minutes, stirring halfway through, until golden brown.
- Remove from the oven and let cool. Stir in the dried fruit.

Granola is a powerhouse of fiber and healthy fats, making it a nutrient-dense food that keeps you full longer. The oats and nuts in granola help reduce cholesterol levels and improve gut health, making it a heart-healthy choice.

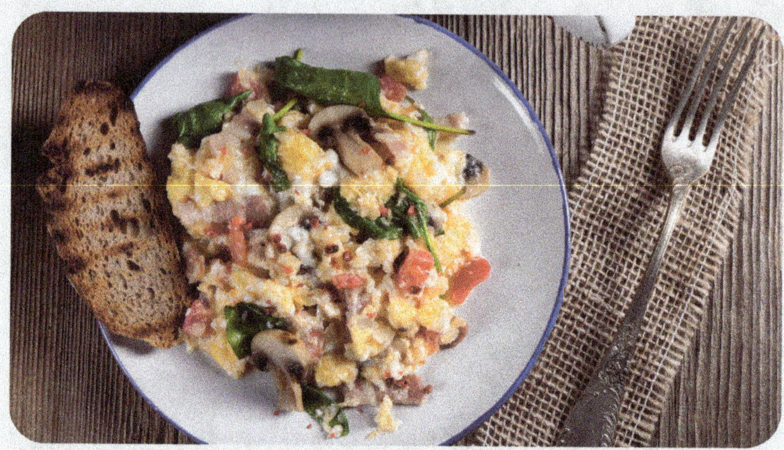

# SCRAMBLED EGGS WITH BASIL, SPINACH & TOMATOES

## Ingredients:

- 2 eggs
- 1/2 cup fresh spinach, chopped
- 1/4 cup cherry tomatoes, halved
- 1 tbsp fresh basil, chopped
- 1 tbsp olive oil
- Salt and pepper to taste

## Instructions:

- Heat olive oil in a skillet over medium heat.
- Add the spinach and tomatoes, and cook until the spinach is wilted.
- Beat the eggs in a bowl and pour into the skillet.
- Stir gently until the eggs are cooked through.
- Sprinkle with basil, salt, and pepper before serving.

This dish is brimming with vitamins and antioxidants from the fresh veggies and herbs. Spinach is rich in iron and fiber, while tomatoes provide a good dose of vitamin C, making this a supercharged breakfast for overall health.

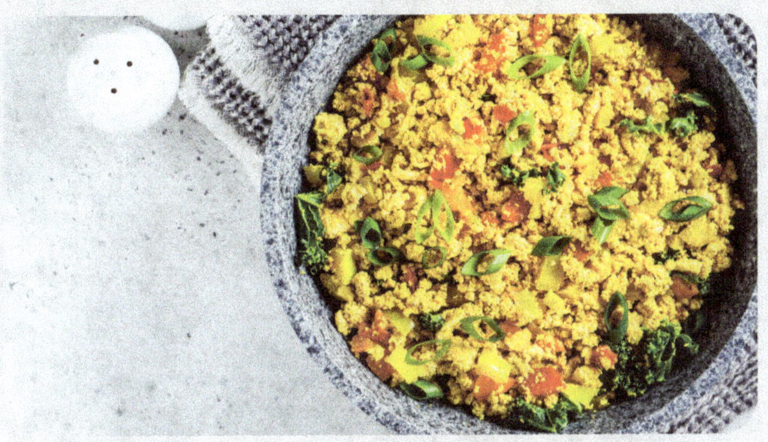

# TOFU SCRAMBLE

## Ingredients:

- 1 block firm tofu, crumbled
- 1/2 cup cherry tomatoes, halved
- 1/4 cup diced bell pepper
- 1/4 cup diced onion
- 1 tbsp olive oil
- 1 tsp turmeric
- Salt and pepper to taste

## Instructions:

- Heat olive oil in a skillet over medium heat.
- Add the onion and bell pepper, and cook until softened.
- Add the crumbled tofu and turmeric, and cook for 5-7 minutes.
- Stir in the cherry tomatoes and cook for another 2 minutes.
- Season with salt and pepper before serving.

A protein-packed, cholesterol-free alternative to scrambled eggs, tofu scramble is also high in calcium and iron. The addition of turmeric not only adds flavor but also provides anti-inflammatory benefits.

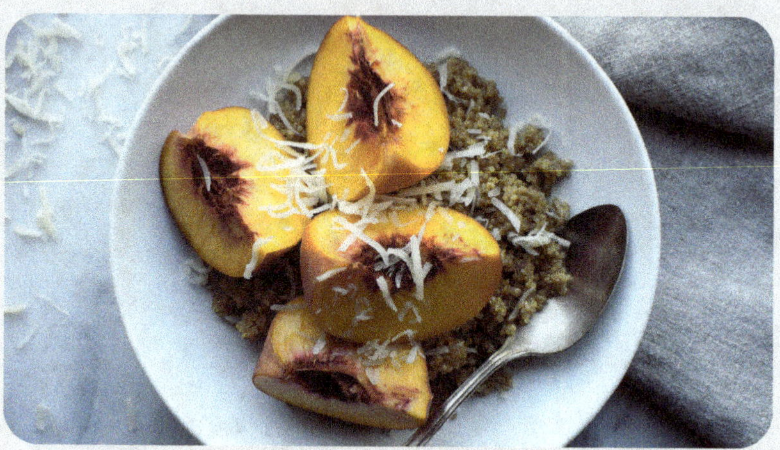

# CARDAMOM & PEACH QUINOA PORRIDGE

## Ingredients:

- 1/2 cup quinoa, rinsed
- 1 cup almond milk
- 1 ripe peach, sliced
- 1/2 tsp ground cardamom
- 1 tbsp honey or maple syrup

## Instructions:

- In a saucepan, combine quinoa, almond milk, and cardamom.
- Bring to a boil, then reduce heat and simmer for 15 minutes, or until quinoa is tender.
- Stir in the honey or maple syrup.
- Serve topped with sliced peach.

Quinoa is a complete protein, while peaches provide vitamin C and antioxidants. This porridge is a perfect blend of flavors and nutrients, making it a great start to your day.

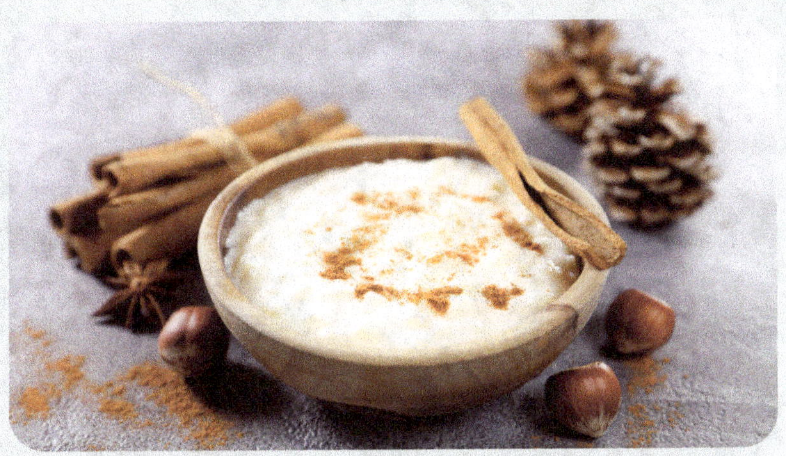

# VANILLA & CINNAMON BREAKFAST RICE

## Ingredients:

- 1 cup cooked brown rice
- 1 cup almond milk
- 1/2 tsp vanilla extract
- 1/2 tsp ground cinnamon
- 1/4 cup chopped dried apricots
- 1/4 cup chopped walnuts almond milk
- 1 ripe peach, sliced
- 1/2 tsp ground cardamom
- 1 tbsp honey or maple syrup

## Instructions:

- In a saucepan, combine cooked rice, almond milk, vanilla extract, and cinnamon.
- Heat over medium heat until warm.
- Stir in the dried apricots and walnuts.
- Serve immediately.

Brown rice offers fiber and the cinnamon helps stabilize blood sugar levels. This comforting breakfast dish is also rich in antioxidants and can keep you full and satisfied throughout the morning.

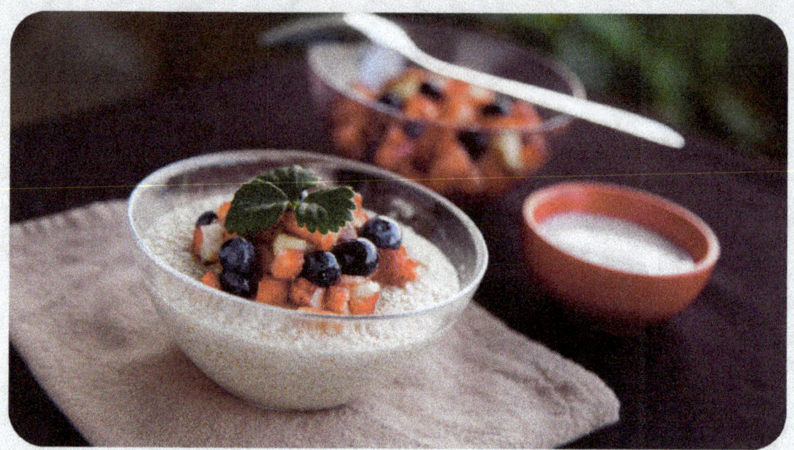

# STRAWBERRY & BLUEBERRY BIRCHER

## Ingredients:

- 1 cup rolled oats
- 1 cup almond milk
- 1/2 cup fresh blueberries
- 1 orange, peeled and segmented
- 1 tbsp chia seeds
- 1 tbsp honey

## Instructions:

- In a bowl, combine oats, almond milk, chia seeds, and honey.
- Cover and refrigerate overnight.
- In the morning, stir in the blueberries and orange segments.
- Serve chilled.

The berries are loaded with antioxidants and the oats give you long-lasting energy. This refreshing breakfast is also high in fiber, which aids in digestion and keeps you feeling full.

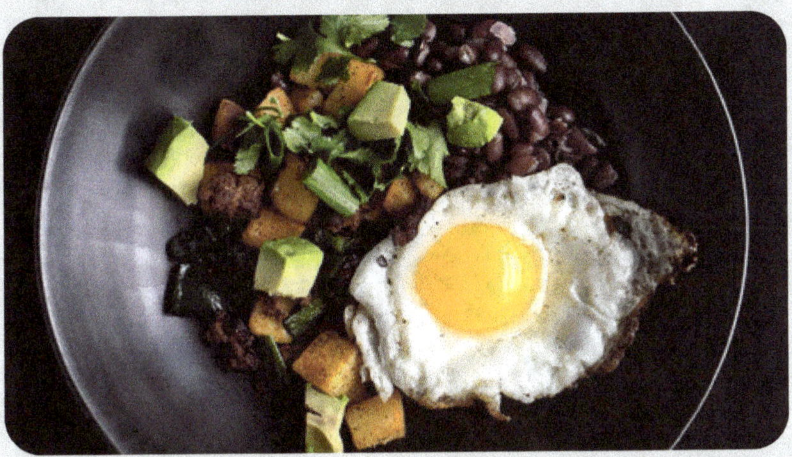

# AVOCADO & BLACK BEAN EGGS

## Ingredients:

- 2 eggs
- 1/2 avocado, sliced
- 1/4 cup black beans, rinsed and drained
- 1 tbsp olive oil
- Salt and pepper to taste

## Instructions:

- Heat olive oil in a skillet over medium heat.
- Crack the eggs into the skillet and cook to your desired doneness.
- Top with avocado slices and black beans.
- Season with salt and pepper before serving.

Avocados provide healthy fats that support heart health, while black beans add fiber and protein. This combination makes for a nutrient-dense and satisfying breakfast.

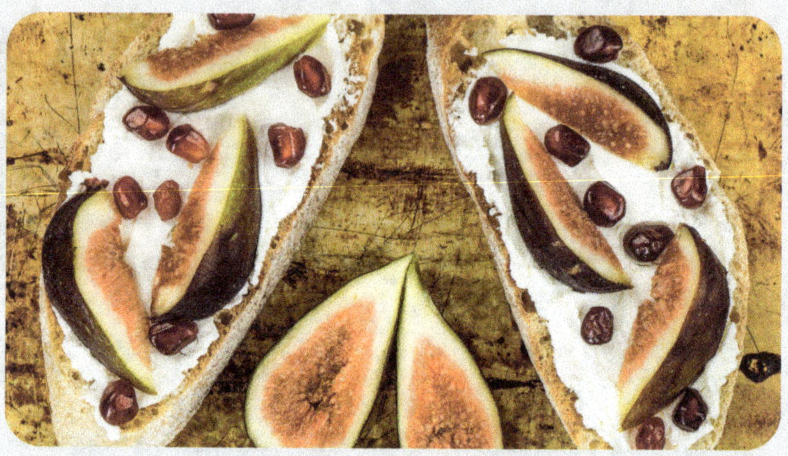

# FIG, NUT & SEED BREAD WITH RICOTTA & FRUIT

## Ingredients:

- 2 slices fig, nut, and seed bread
- 1/4 cup ricotta cheese
- 1/2 apple or orange, sliced

## Instructions:

- Toast the bread slices.
- Spread ricotta cheese on each slice.
- Top with apple or orange slices.
- Serve immediately.

Packed with nutrients from figs, nuts, seeds, and ricotta cheese, this breakfast is a delicious way to start your day with a boost of protein, fiber, and healthy fats.

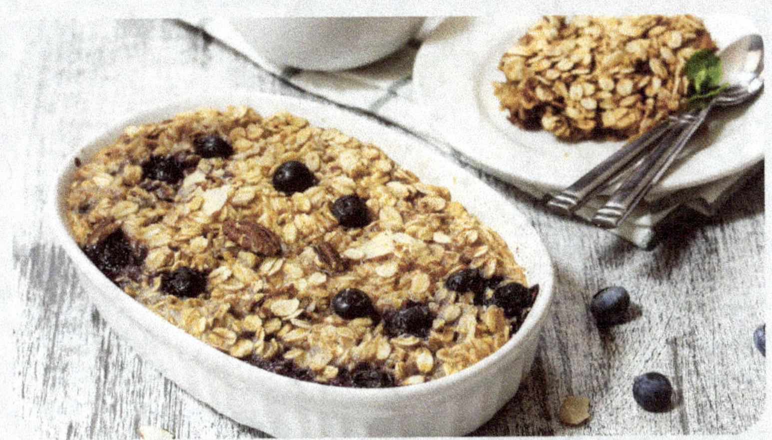

# BLUEBERRY BAKED OATS

## Ingredients:

- 1 cup rolled oats
- 1 cup almond milk
- 1/2 cup fresh blueberries
- 1/4 cup chopped almonds
- 1 tbsp honey
- 1/2 tsp vanilla extract

## Instructions:

- Preheat the oven to 350°F (175°C).
- In a bowl, combine oats, almond milk, honey, and vanilla extract.
- Stir in the blueberries and almonds.
- Pour the mixture into a baking dish.
- Bake for 25-30 minutes, or until golden brown.
- Serve warm.

**Blueberries are antioxidant powerhouses and oats release energy slowly, making this a perfect breakfast to keep you energized and focused throughout the morning.**

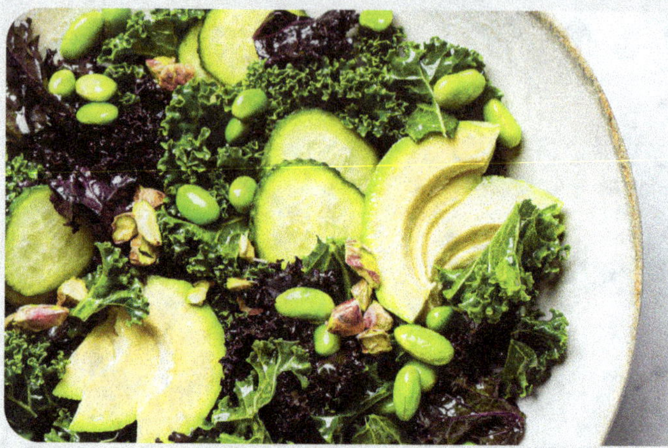

# SMASHED CUCUMBER & EDAMAME

## Ingredients:

- 1 cucumber, smashed and sliced
- 1/2 cup edamame, shelled
- 1 tbsp soy sauce
- 1 tsp sesame oil
- 1 tsp rice vinegar

## Instructions:

- In a bowl, combine soy sauce, sesame oil, and rice vinegar.
- Add the cucumber and edamame, and toss to coat.
- Garnish with sesame seeds and cilantro before serving.

Edamame provides plant-based protein and the cucumber is hydrating. This refreshing snack is also rich in antioxidants and fiber, promoting overall health.

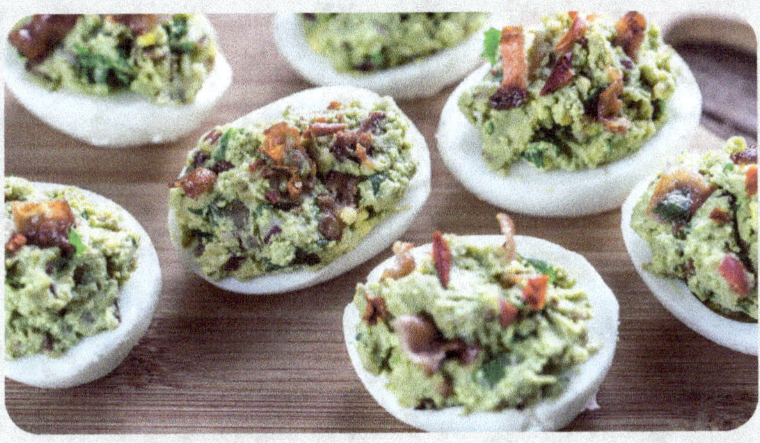

# AVOCADO DEVILED EGGS

## Ingredients:

- 4 hard-boiled eggs, halved
- 1/2 avocado, mashed
- 1 tbsp Greek yogurt
- 1 tsp lemon juice
- Salt and pepper to taste

## Instructions:

- Remove the yolks from the hard-boiled eggs and place them in a bowl.
- Add the mashed avocado, Greek yogurt, lemon juice, salt, and pepper.
- Mix until smooth.
- Spoon the mixture back into the egg whites.
- Serve immediately.

Avocado lends healthy fats and the eggs are a great source of protein. This combination makes for a nutrient-dense snack that supports muscle repair and heart health.

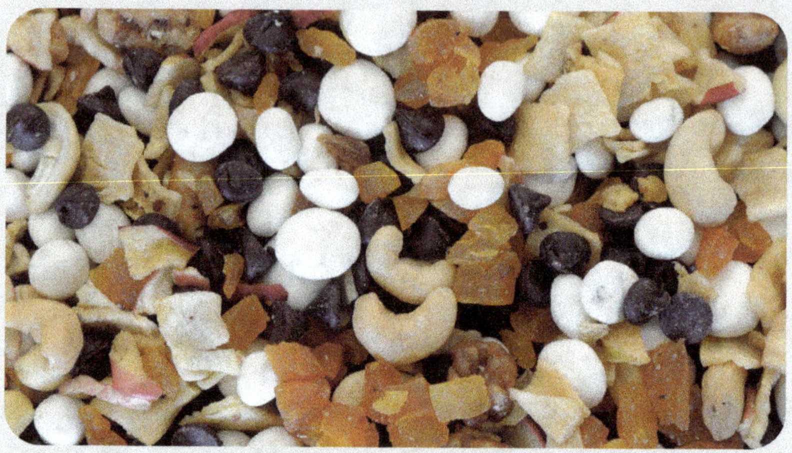

# CINNAMON & APRICOT TRAIL MIX

## Ingredients:

- 1 cup mixed nuts (almonds, walnuts, pecans)
- 1/2 cup dried apricots, chopped
- 1/4 cup pumpkin seeds
- 1/4 cup sunflower seeds
- 1 tsp ground cinnamon

## Instructions:

- In a bowl, combine all ingredients.
- Store in an airtight container.
- Enjoy as a snack throughout the day.

Cinnamon has anti-inflammatory benefits and the nuts/seeds provide protein and healthy fats. This trail mix is a perfect on-the-go snack that supports heart health and keeps you energized.

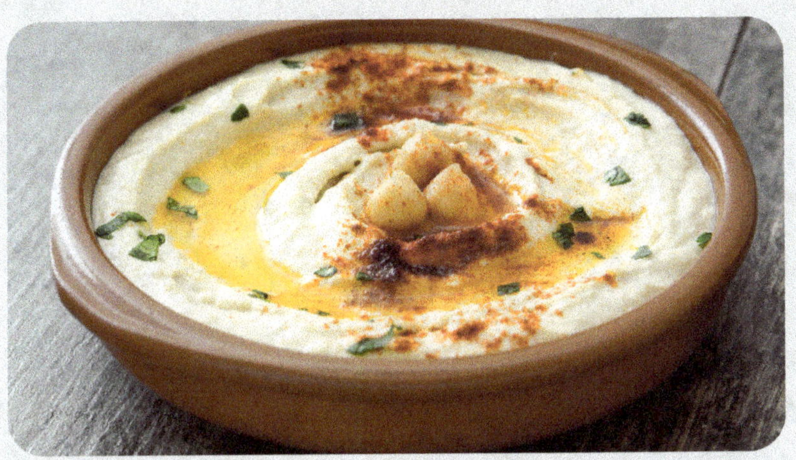

# CHICKPEA & RED PEPPER DIP

## Ingredients:

- 1 can chickpeas, drained and rinsed
- 1 red bell pepper, roasted and chopped
- 1 clove garlic, minced
- 2 tbsp olive oil
- 1 tbsp lemon juice
- Salt and pepper to taste

## Instructions:

- In a food processor, combine chickpeas, red bell pepper, garlic, olive oil, and lemon juice.
- Blend until smooth.
- Season with salt and pepper.
- Serve with vegetable sticks or whole-grain crackers.

Chickpeas offer protein and fiber while red peppers are packed with vitamin C. This dip is a delicious and nutritious snack that supports immune health and digestion.

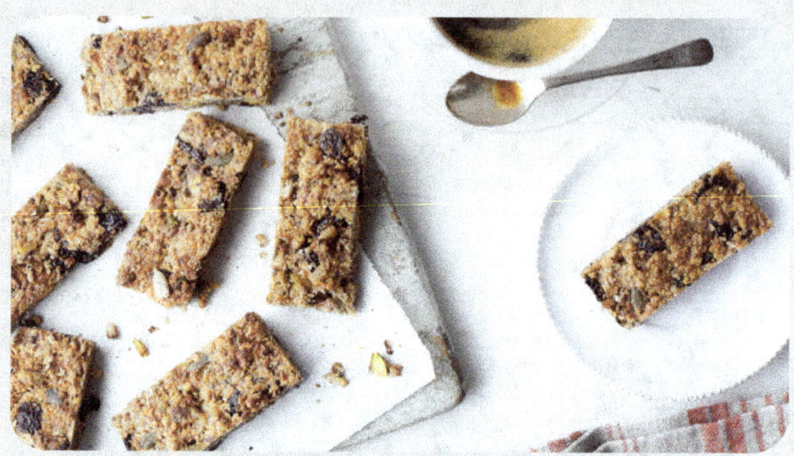

# HEALTHY FLAPJACKS

## Ingredients:

- 2 cups rolled oats
- 1/2 cup chopped dates
- 1/4 cup chopped walnuts
- 1/4 cup honey or maple syrup
- 1/4 cup coconut oil, melted

## Instructions:

- Preheat the oven to 350°F (175°C).
- In a bowl, combine oats, dates, walnuts, honey, and coconut oil.
- Press the mixture into a baking dish.
- Bake for 20-25 minutes, or until golden brown.
- Let cool before cutting into bars.

Made with oats and fruit for fiber and natural sweetness without refined sugar, these flapjacks are a healthy and satisfying snack that supports digestive health and provides lasting energy.

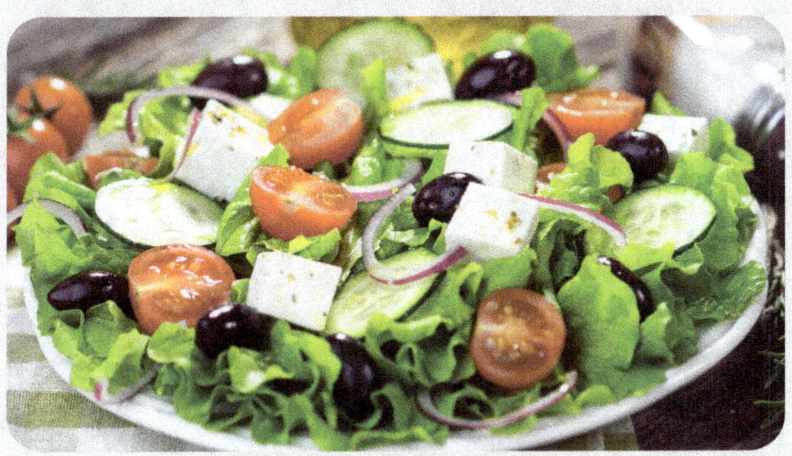

# GREEK SALAD

## Ingredients:

- 1 English cucumber and 1 green bell pepper
- 2 cups halved cherry tomatoes
- 5 ounces feta cheese
- ⅓ cup thinly sliced red onion and olives
- ⅓ cup fresh mint leaves
- ¼ cup extra-virgin olive oil
- 3 tablespoons red wine vinegar
- 1 garlic clove, minced
- dried oregano, Dijon mustard, sea salt and freshly ground black pepper

## Instructions:

- In a small bowl, whisk together the olive oil, vinegar, garlic, oregano, mustard, salt, and several grinds of pepper.
- On a large platter, arrange the cucumber, green pepper, cherry tomatoes, feta cheese, red onions, and olives.
- Drizzle with the dressing and very gently toss.
- Sprinkle with a few generous pinches of oregano and top with the mint leaves. Season to taste and serve.

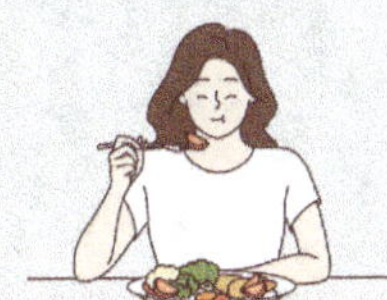

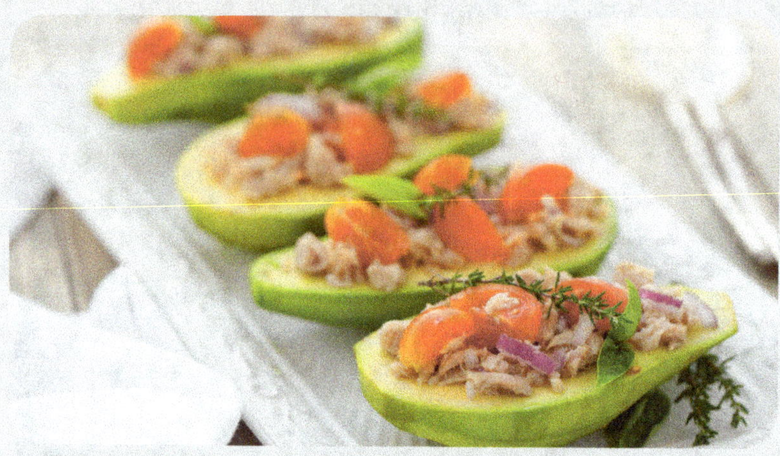

# TUNA STUFFED AVOCADO

## Ingredients:

- 4 avocados
- 2 (5 oz) cans tuna, drained
- 1/4 cup mayonnaise
- 1 stalk of celery, diced
- 2 tbsp red onion, diced
- 1-2 tbsp chopped parsley, chives, and/or other herbs
- 1/2 tbsp Dijon mustard
- Salt and pepper to taste

## Instructions:

- In a mixing bowl, combine tuna, mayonnaise, celery, red onion, herbs, Dijon mustard, salt, and pepper. Stir together until well combined.
- Slice the avocados in half and remove the seed.
- Dollop a few spoonfuls of tuna salad onto each avocado half.

Tuna is high in protein and avocado lends heart-healthy fats. This combination makes for a satisfying and nutritious meal that supports muscle repair and heart health.

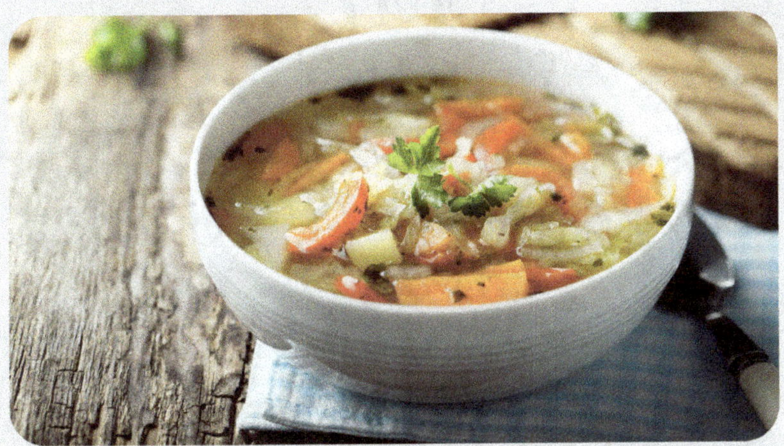

# VEGETABLE SOUP

---

### Ingredients:

- 2 Tbsp olive oil
- 1 1/2 cups chopped yellow onion
- 2 cups carrots (about 5)
- 1/4 cups chopped celery
- 4 cloves garlic, minced
- 4 (14.5 oz) cans chicken broth or vegetable broth
- 2 diced tomatoes
- 3 cups diced potatoes
- 1/3 cup fresh parsley
- 2 bay leaves
- 1/2 tsp dried thyme
- Salt and black pepper
- 1 1/2 cups green beans
- 1 1/4 cups frozen or fresh corn
- 1 cup frozen or fresh peas

### Instructions:

- Heat olive oil in a large pot over medium-high heat.
- Add onions, carrots, and celery and sauté for 4 minutes, then add garlic and sauté for 30 seconds longer.
- Add in broth, tomatoes, potatoes, parsley, bay leaves, thyme, and season with salt and pepper to taste.
- Bring to a boil, then add green beans.
- Reduce heat to medium-low, cover, and simmer until potatoes are almost fully tender, about 20-30 minutes.
- Add corn and peas and cook for 5 minutes longer. Serve warm.

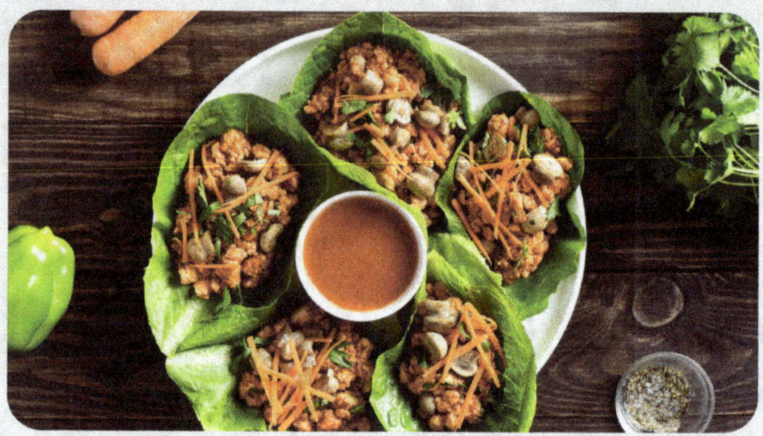

# TURKEY LETTUCE WRAPS

## Ingredients:

- 2 Tbsp olive oil
- 1 lb lean ground turkey
- 1 tbsp olive oil
- 1/2 cup diced onion
- 1/2 cup diced bell pepper
- 2 cloves garlic, minced
- 1 tbsp soy sauce
- 1 tbsp hoisin sauce
- 1 tbsp rice vinegar
- 1 tsp roasted red chili paste
- 1/4 cup chopped green onions
- 1/4 cup chopped water chestnuts
- Bibb lettuce leaves

## Instructions:

- Heat olive oil in a large skillet over medium-high heat. Add turkey, garlic, and ginger to the pan and cook for about 6 minutes.
- While the turkey is cooking, whisk together hoisin, soy sauce, rice vinegar, and roasted red chili paste in a small bowl.
- Once the ground turkey is cooked through, turn the heat off and add in the chopped green onions and water chestnuts. Drizzle with sauce and stir well until coated completely.
- Spoon about a ¼ cup of the turkey mixture onto each lettuce leaf. Serve warm.

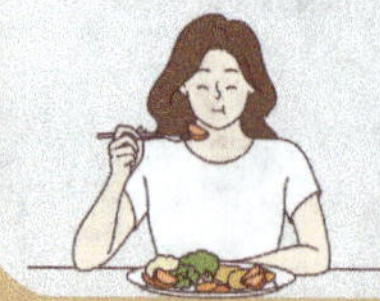

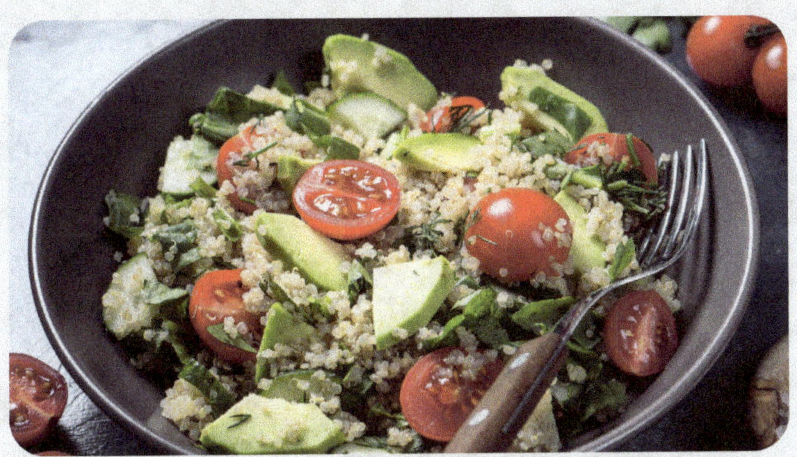

# QUINOA VEGGIE SALAD

## Ingredients:

- 1 cup cooked quinoa
- 1 cup cherry tomatoes, halved
- 1 cucumber, diced
- 1/2 red onion, diced
- 1/2 cup diced bell pepper
- 1/4 cup chopped parsley
- 1/4 cup olive oil
- 2 tbsp lemon juice
- Salt and pepper to taste
- Bibb lettuce leaves

## Instructions:

- In a large bowl, combine cooked quinoa, cherry tomatoes, cucumber, red onion, bell pepper, and parsley.
- In a small bowl, whisk together olive oil, lemon juice, salt, and pepper.
- Pour dressing over quinoa salad and toss to coat.

Quinoa is a complete protein and the veggies add fiber, vitamins, and minerals. This salad is a nutrient-dense meal that supports overall health and keeps you full and satisfied.

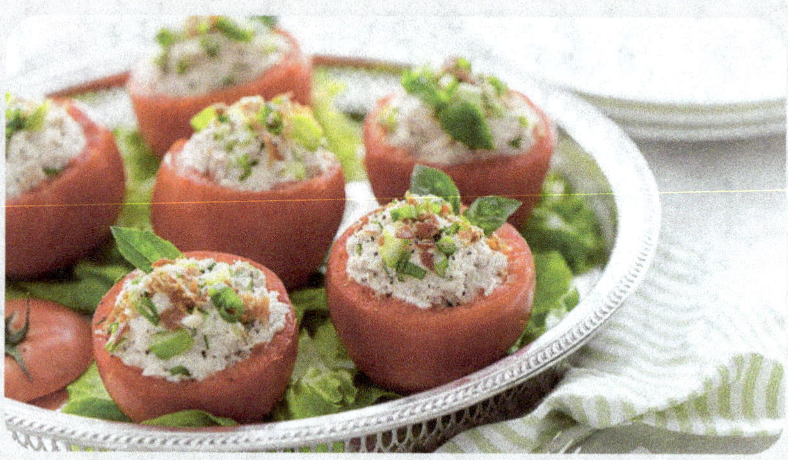

# CHICKEN SALAD STUFFED TOMATOES

## Ingredients:

- 3 cups cooked and shredded chicken
- 1 cup chopped celery
- 1/4 cup chopped green onion
- 3/4 cup mayonnaise
- 1 tbsp lemon juice
- 1/2 tsp salt
- 1/2 tsp black pepper
- 1/2 tsp onion powder
- 1/4 tsp garlic powder
- 8 large tomatoes

## Instructions:

- In a large mixing bowl, combine chicken, celery, green onion, mayonnaise, lemon juice, salt, pepper, onion powder, and garlic powder. Stir until combined well. Refrigerate until ready to serve.
- Using a sharp knife, cut the top of large, ripe tomatoes (about 1" down from top) and carefully remove all tomato pulp.
- Take a paper towel and dab inside the tomato to dry up any juices.
- Use an ice cream scoop to scoop your chicken salad into the hollowed-out tomato shell.

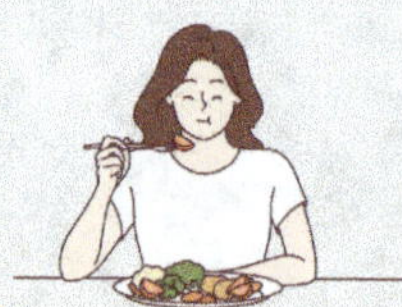

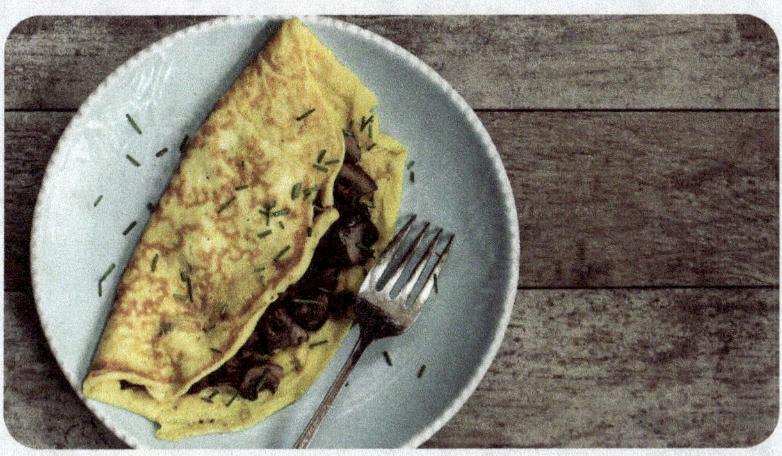

# VEGGIE FRITTATA

## Ingredients:

- 6 large eggs
- 1/4 cup milk
- 1/2 cup chopped spinach
- 1/2 cup sliced mushrooms
- 1/2 cup diced bell pepper
- 1/4 cup crumbled feta cheese
- 1 tbsp olive oil
- Salt and pepper to taste

**Eggs provide protein and the veggies lend fiber, vitamins, and minerals. This frittata is a delicious and nutrient-dense meal that supports overall health and keeps you energized.**

## Instructions:

- Preheat oven to 375°F (190°C).
- In a bowl, whisk together eggs, milk, salt, and pepper.
- Heat olive oil in an oven-safe skillet over medium heat. Add spinach, mushrooms, and bell pepper, and cook until vegetables are tender.
- Pour egg mixture over the vegetables and cook until the edges start to set.
- Sprinkle feta cheese on top and transfer the skillet to the oven.
- Bake for 10-15 minutes, or until the frittata is fully set and slightly golden on top.

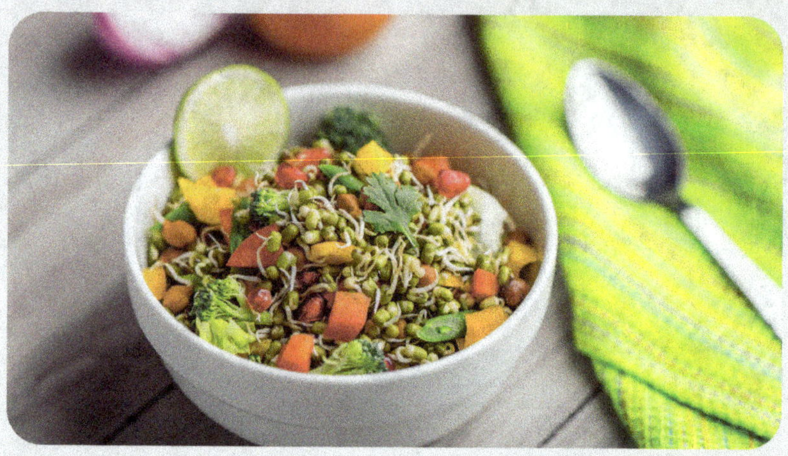

# LENTIL SALAD

---

## Ingredients:

- 1 cup cooked lentils
- 1/2 cup diced cucumber
- 1/2 cup diced bell pepper
- 1/4 cup diced red onion
- 1/4 cup crumbled feta cheese
- 2 tbsp chopped fresh dill
- 2 tbsp olive oil
- 1 tbsp lemon juice
- Salt and pepper to taste

## Instructions:

- In a large bowl, combine cooked lentils, cucumber, bell pepper, red onion, feta cheese, and dill.
- In a small bowl, whisk together olive oil, lemon juice, salt, and pepper.
- Pour dressing over lentil salad and toss to coat.

Lentils are high in protein and fiber to keep you satisfied. This salad is a nutritious and filling meal that supports digestive health and muscle repair.

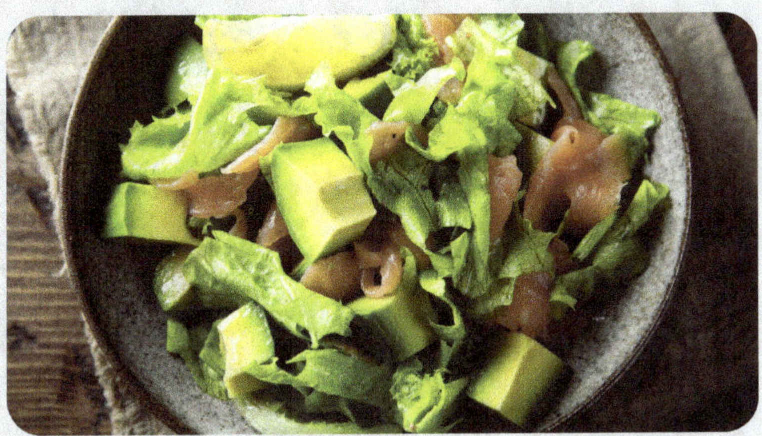

# SALMON AVOCADO SALAD

## Ingredients:

- 4 cups mixed greens
- 1 baked salmon fillet, flaked
- 1 avocado, sliced
- 1 cup cherry tomatoes, halved
- 1 cucumber, sliced
- 1/4 cup balsamic vinaigrette

## Instructions:

- In a large bowl, combine mixed greens, flaked salmon, avocado, cherry tomatoes, and cucumber.
- Drizzle with balsamic vinaigrette and toss gently to combine.

Salmon is high in omega-3s and avocado provides heart-healthy fats. This salad is a delicious and nutrient-dense meal that supports heart health and brain function.

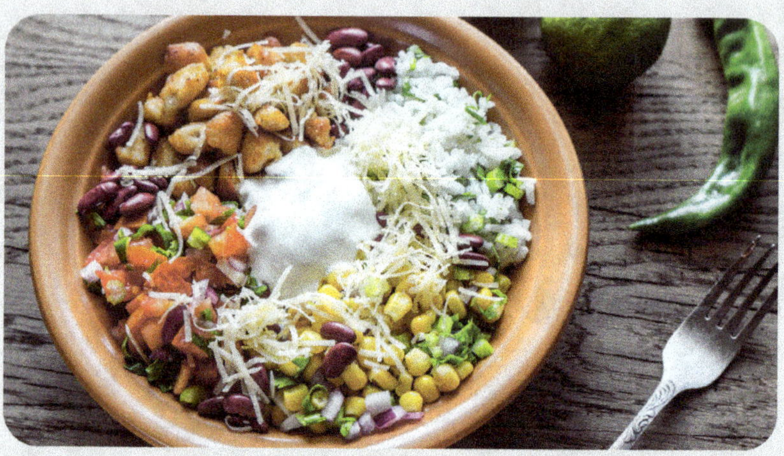

# CAULIFLOWER RICE BURRITO BOWL

## Ingredients:

- 2 cups cauliflower rice
- 1 can black beans, rinsed and drained
- 1 cup pico de gallo
- 1 avocado, sliced
- 1/4 cup Greek yogurt
- 1 tbsp lime juice
- Fresh cilantro for garnish

## Instructions:

- Cook cauliflower rice according to package instructions.
- In a bowl, layer cauliflower rice, black beans, pico de gallo, and avocado slices.
- Top with a dollop of Greek yogurt and a drizzle of lime juice.
- Garnish with fresh cilantro before serving.

Cauliflower rice is low-carb but high in fiber and antioxidants. This burrito bowl is a healthy and satisfying meal that supports digestive health and weight management.

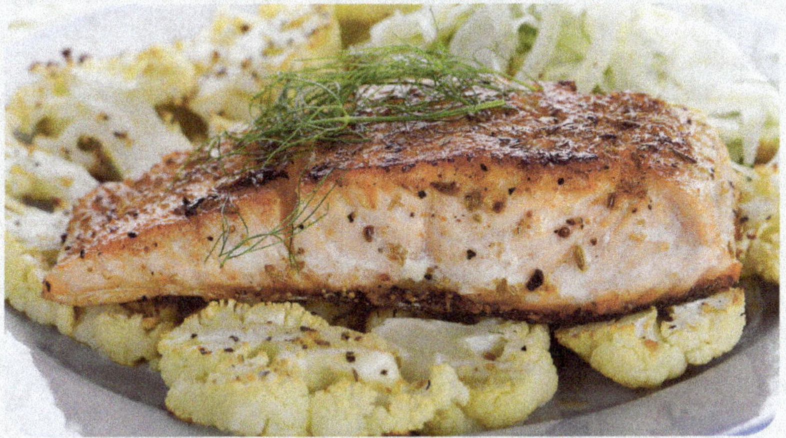

# BAKED SALMON WITH ROASTED VEGGIES

## Ingredients:

- 4 (6 oz) salmon fillets
- 2 cups broccoli florets
- 2 cups cauliflower florets
- 2 tbsp olive oil, divided
- 1 lemon, sliced
- Salt, pepper, garlic powder to taste

**Salmon is high in omega-3s and the veggies provide fiber and vitamins. This meal is a delicious and nutrient-dense option that supports heart health and overall well-being.**

## Instructions:

- Preheat oven to 400°F (200°C). Line a baking sheet with foil.
- Toss broccoli and cauliflower with 1 tbsp olive oil and season with salt and pepper. Spread on one side of the baking sheet.
- Place salmon fillets on the other side and brush with remaining 1 tbsp olive oil. Season with salt, pepper, and garlic powder.
- Top salmon with lemon slices.
- Roast for 15-20 minutes until salmon is opaque and veggies are tender.

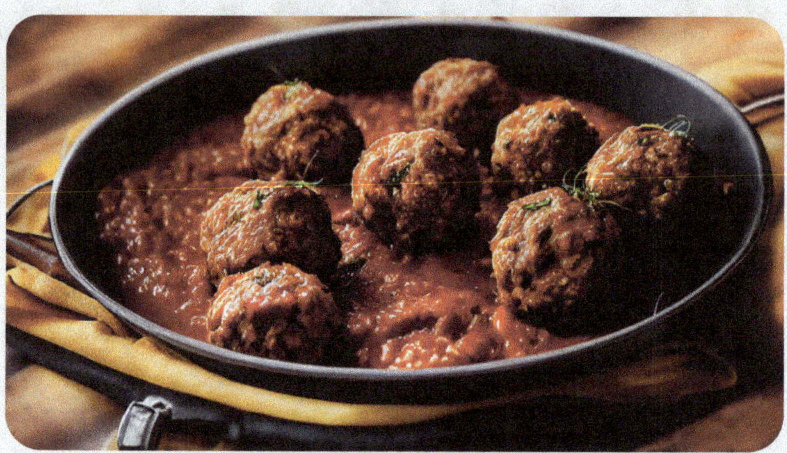

# TURKEY QUINOA MEATBALLS

## Ingredients:

- 1 lb ground turkey
- 1 cup cooked quinoa
- 1 egg
- 1/2 cup breadcrumbs
- 1/4 cup grated parmesan
- 1/4 cup parsley, chopped
- 2 cloves garlic, minced
- 1 tsp Italian seasoning
- Salt and pepper to taste
- 1 jar marinara sauce

Lean turkey and quinoa make these meatballs a protein powerhouse. This meal is a delicious and nutritious option that supports muscle repair and weight management.

## Instructions:

- Preheat oven to 400°F (200°C). Lightly grease a baking sheet.
- In a bowl, mix together turkey, quinoa, egg, breadcrumbs, parmesan, parsley, garlic, Italian seasoning, and salt & pepper until well combined.
- Form mixture into 1-inch meatballs and place on prepared baking sheet.
- Bake for 15-18 minutes until cooked through.
- Serve meatballs over whole wheat pasta or zucchini noodles with marinara sauce.

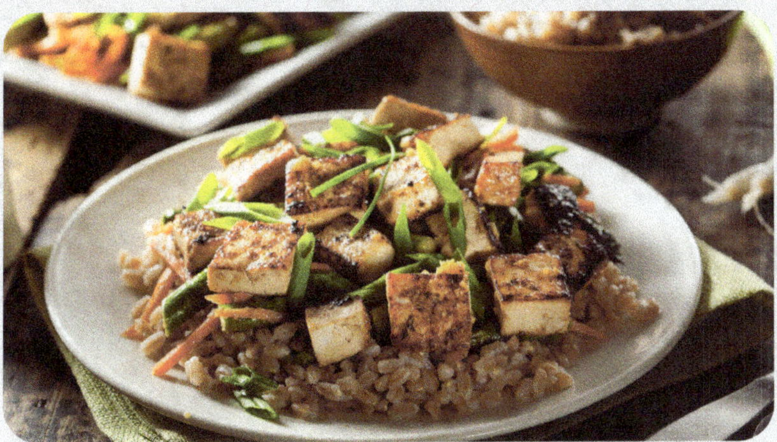

# VEGETABLE STIR FRY

---

### Ingredients:

- 2 tbsp olive oil
- 1 cup broccoli florets
- 1 cup snap peas
- 1 cup sliced mushrooms
- 1 bell pepper, sliced
- 1 carrot, julienned
- 2 cloves garlic, minced
- 1 tbsp soy sauce
- 1 tbsp hoisin sauce
- 1 tsp grated ginger
- Cooked brown rice

### Instructions:

- Heat olive oil in a wok or large skillet over medium-high heat.
- Add garlic and ginger, and sauté for 30 seconds.
- Add broccoli, snap peas, mushrooms, bell pepper, and carrot. Stir-fry for 5-7 minutes until vegetables are tender-crisp.
- Stir in soy sauce and hoisin sauce, and cook for another 2 minutes.
- Serve over cooked brown rice.

Loaded with fiber and antioxidants from the fresh veggies, this stir fry is a healthy and satisfying meal that supports digestive health and boosts the immune system.

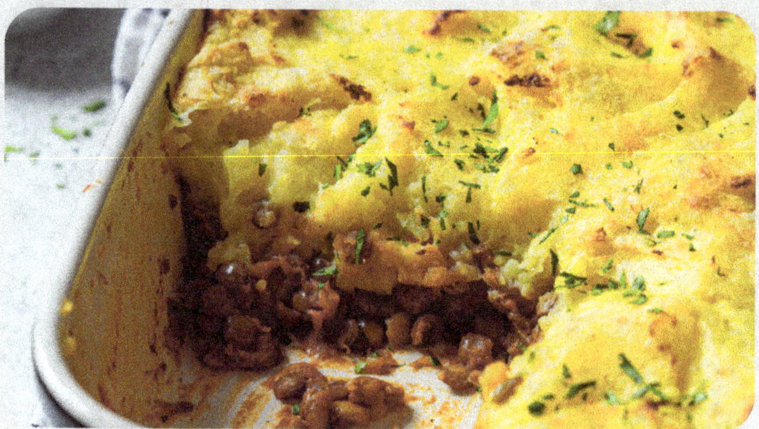

# LENTIL SHEPHERD'S PIE

---

### Ingredients:

- 1 cup cooked lentils
- 1 sweet potato, peeled and mashed
- 1/2 cup diced carrots
- 1/2 cup peas
- 1/4 cup diced onion
- 1 tbsp olive oil
- 1 tsp thyme
- Salt and pepper to taste

### Instructions:

- Preheat oven to 375°F (190°C).
- In a skillet, heat olive oil over medium heat.
- Add diced onion, carrots, and peas, and cook until softened.
- Stir in cooked lentils and thyme, and season with salt and pepper.
- Transfer lentil mixture to a baking dish and spread mashed sweet potato on top.
- Bake for 20-25 minutes until the top is slightly golden.

Lentils provide protein and fiber while veggies add nutrients. This comforting meal is a nutritious and filling option that supports digestive health and muscle repair.

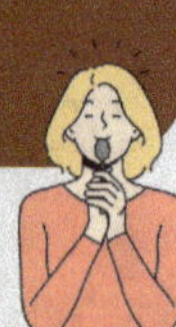

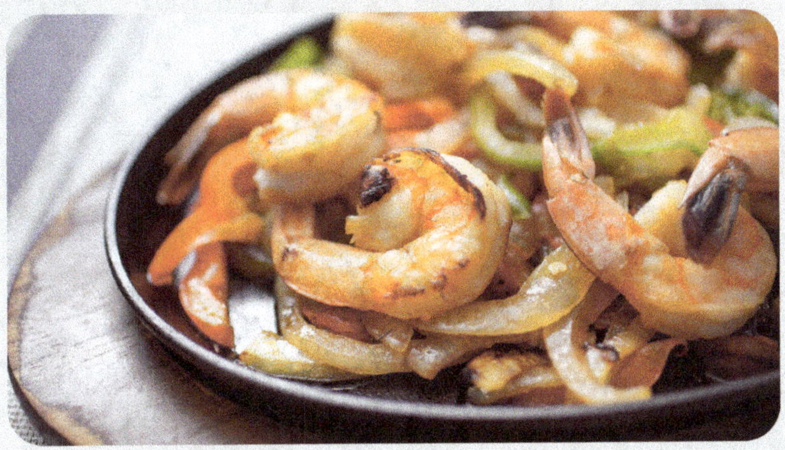

# SHRIMP FAJITAS

---

### Ingredients:

- 1 lb shrimp, peeled and deveined
- 1 bell pepper, sliced
- 1 onion, sliced
- 1 tbsp olive oil
- 1 tsp chili powder
- 1 tsp cumin
- 1/2 tsp paprika
- Salt and pepper to taste
- Lettuce leaves
- Salsa, avocado, and Greek yogurt for serving

### Instructions:

- In a bowl, toss shrimp with chili powder, cumin, paprika, salt, and pepper.
- Heat olive oil in a skillet over medium-high heat.
- Add bell pepper and onion, and cook until softened.
- Add shrimp and cook until pink and opaque.
- Serve shrimp and vegetables in lettuce leaves with salsa, avocado, and Greek yogurt.

Shrimp is low-calorie but high in protein and the veggies offer fiber. This meal is a delicious and healthy option that supports muscle repair and weight management.

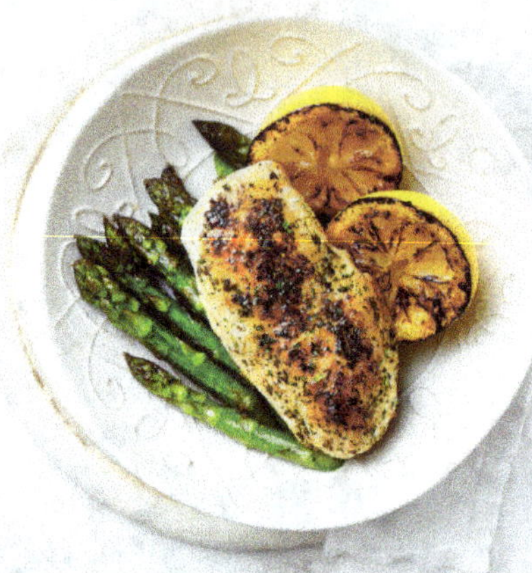

# GRILLED LEMON HERB CHICKEN WITH ASPARAGUS

## Ingredients:

- 4 boneless, skinless chicken breasts
- 2 tablespoons olive oil
- 2 tablespoons lemon juice
- 2 cloves garlic, minced
- 1 teaspoon dried oregano
- 1 teaspoon dried thyme
- Salt and pepper to taste
- 1 bunch asparagus, trimmed
- Lemon wedges for serving

Lean protein from the chicken and fiber from asparagus make this meal a nutritious and satisfying option that supports muscle repair and digestive health.

## Instructions:

- In a small bowl, whisk together olive oil, lemon juice, garlic, oregano, thyme, salt, and pepper.
- Place chicken breasts in a plastic bag and pour the marinade over them. Seal the bag and refrigerate for at least 30 minutes.
- Preheat the grill to medium-high heat.
- Remove chicken from the marinade and grill for 6-7 minutes per side, or until fully cooked.
- While the chicken is grilling, toss asparagus with a little olive oil, salt, and pepper.
- Grill asparagus for 3-4 minutes Serve chicken with grilled asparagus and lemon wedges.

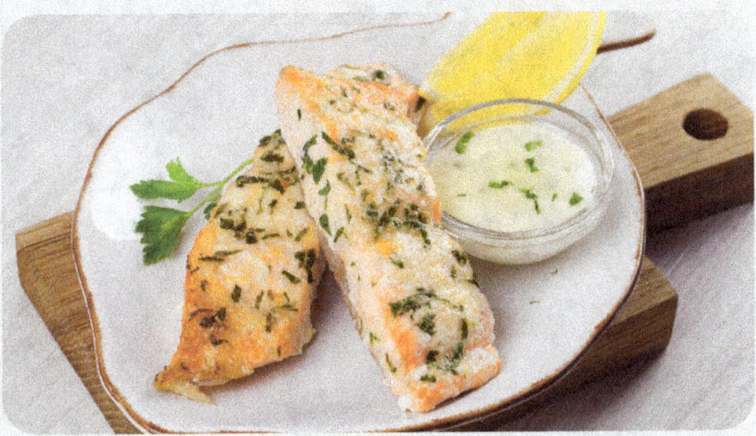

# BAKED COD WITH LEMON AND DILL

## Ingredients:

- 4 cod fillets
- 2 tablespoons olive oil
- 2 tablespoons lemon juice
- 1 tablespoon fresh dill, chopped
- 2 cloves garlic, minced
- Salt and pepper to taste
- Lemon slices for garnish

## Instructions:

- Preheat the oven to 400°F (200°C).
- In a small bowl, mix together olive oil, lemon juice, dill, garlic, salt, and pepper.
- Place cod fillets in a baking dish and brush with the lemon-dill mixture.
- Bake for 12-15 minutes, or until the fish is opaque and flakes easily with a fork.
- Garnish with lemon slices and serve with a side of steamed vegetables.

Cod is high in protein and low in calories and fat. This meal is a delicious and healthy option that supports muscle repair and weight management.

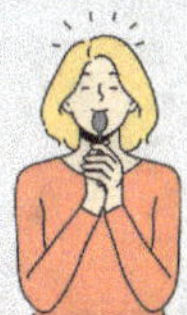

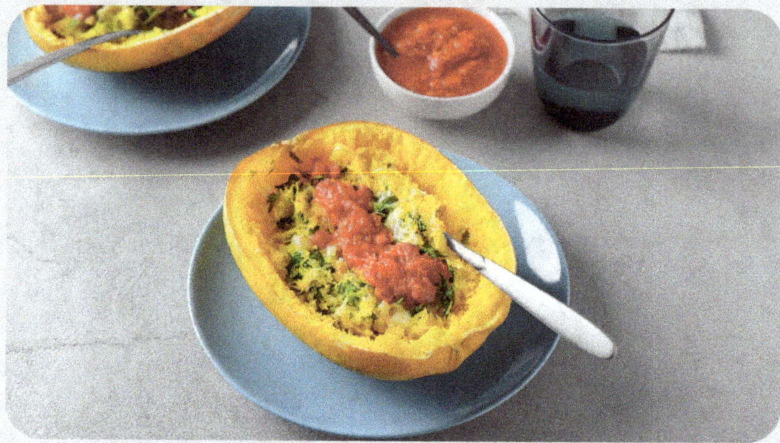

# SPAGHETTI SQUASH PRIMAVERA

## Ingredients:

- 1 large spaghetti squash
- 2 tablespoons olive oil
- 1 cup cherry tomatoes, halved
- 1 zucchini, diced
- 1 yellow squash, diced
- 1 red bell pepper, diced
- 2 cloves garlic, minced
- 1/4 cup grated Parmesan cheese
- Fresh basil for garnish

Spaghetti squash is low-carb and the veggies provide fiber and antioxidants. This meal is a healthy and satisfying option that supports digestive health and weight management.

## Instructions:

- Preheat the oven to 400°
- Cut the spaghetti squash and scoop out the seeds. Drizzle with 1 tablespoon olive oil and season with salt and pepper.
- Place the squash halves on a baking sheet and roast for 40-45 minutes
- Heat the remaining olive oil in a large skillet and add garlic
- Add cherry tomatoes, zucchini, yellow squash, and bell pepper. Cook for 5-7 minutes.
- Once the squash is done, use a fork to scrape out the spaghetti-like strands into a large bowl.
- Add the cooked vegetables to the bowl and toss to combine.

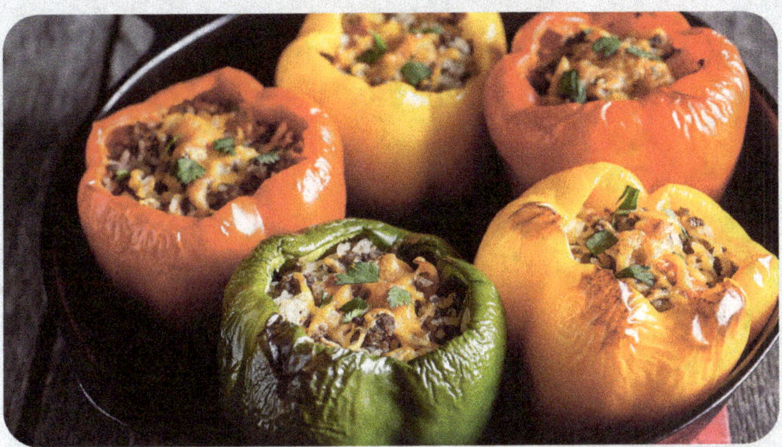

# STUFFED BELL PEPPERS

---

### Ingredients:

- 4 large bell peppers, tops cut off and seeds removed
- 1 cup cooked quinoa
- 1 can (15 oz) black beans, drained and rinsed
- 1 cup corn kernels
- 1 cup diced tomatoes
- 1/2 cup shredded cheddar cheese
- 1 teaspoon cumin
- 1 teaspoon chili powder
- Salt and pepper to taste
- Fresh cilantro for garnish

This dip is a delicious and nutritious snack that supports*health and muscle repair.

### Instructions:

- Preheat the oven to 375°F (190°C).
- In a large bowl, combine cooked quinoa, black beans, corn, diced tomatoes, cumin, chili powder, salt, and pepper.
- Stuff each bell pepper with the quinoa mixture and place them in a baking dish.
- Cover the dish with foil and bake for 30 minutes.
- Remove the foil, sprinkle the tops with shredded cheese, and bake for an additional 10 minutes, or until the cheese is melted and the peppers are tender.

Garnish with fresh cilantro before serving.

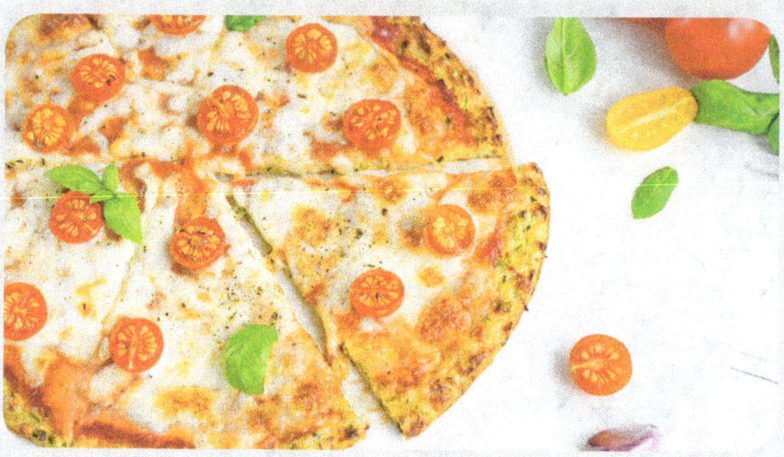

# ZUCCHINI CRUST PIZZA

## Ingredients:

- 2 medium zucchinis, grated
- 1/4 cup grated Parmesan cheese
- 1/4 cup shredded mozzarella cheese
- 1 egg, beaten
- 1/2 teaspoon dried oregano
- 1/2 teaspoon garlic powder
- Salt and pepper to taste
- 1/2 cup marinara sauce
- 1 cup shredded mozzarella cheese (for topping)
- Your favorite pizza toppings

Zucchini makes a nutrient-dense, low-carb pizza crust. This meal is a healthy and satisfying option that supports weight management and overall health.

## Instructions:

- Preheat the oven to 425°
- Place the grated zucchini in a kitchen towel and squeeze out as much moisture as possible.
- Combine the zucchini, Parmesan cheese, 1/4 cup mozzarella cheese, egg, oregano, garlic powder, salt, and pepper.
- Spread the zucchini mixture onto baking sheet, forming a thin crust.
- Bake for 15-20 minutes
- Remove from the oven and spread marinara sauce over the crust. Top with 1 cup shredded mozzarella cheese
- Bake for an additional 10-15 minutes, or until the cheese is melted and bubbly.

www.ingramcontent.com/pod-product-compliance
Lightning Source LLC
Chambersburg PA
CBHW051823250726
48659CB00005B/1640